Fit For Life

Fit For Life

BOOST YOUR HEALTH AND WELLBEING WITH PRACTICAL FITNESS PLANS

Edited by

EMMA VAN HINSBERGH

SIRIUS

SIRIUS

This edition published in 2023 by Sirius Publishing, a division of
Arcturus Publishing Limited,
26/27 Bickels Yard, 151–153 Bermondsey Street,
London SE1 3HA

Copyright © Arcturus Holdings Limited
Text © Kelsey Publishing Limited

ISBN: 978-1-3988-2044-9
AD008850UK

Printed in China

CONTENTS

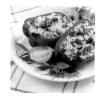

WHY EXERCISE?

How long have you got? There are so many health benefits to being active and they all translate into a healthier, more vibrant you.

Choosing to exercise in a class gives you the benefits of a motivating teacher and the enjoyment of doing it alongside others.

The benefits of being physically active are endless. If you exercise regularly, you will have a reduced risk of coronary heart disease and stroke, better muscular strength and flexibility, reduced risk of type 2 diabetes and obesity, improved balance and coordination and lower levels of stress and anxiety. You will also be more likely to sleep better, which will help you look and feel younger, and you'll be less likely to suffer from depression, as well as having greater self-esteem. Being more physically active can literally add years to your life and it's never too late to start exercising when you want to reap the benefits. Lifestyle is the main contributing factor of premature death so, put simply, if you exercise, you will live longer. If you're currently not exercising, you may be blaming it on many reasons – lack of time, feeling self-conscious or feeling too tired to do anything after a long day at work. Even those who exercise regularly will admit there's always an excuse not to do it if they really want one and there will be days when it's more tempting to stay on the sofa. Some people don't exercise purely because they don't consider themselves 'the sporty type'. But you don't have to be sporty to exercise and you don't need to spend hours and hours doing it to get results. Even small levels of activity can have significant benefits. The recommended guidelines for cardiovascular exercise (such as cycling, running, brisk walking, swimming, or anything similar that raises your heart rate and gets you moderately out of breath) are three to five times per week for 20 to 90 minutes each time. Break this down and it doesn't sound too bad. If you take the lower levels of exercise needed, that's just three times per week for 20 minutes each time. Even these levels offer health benefits and of course help you burn calories, which in turn will help you lose weight.

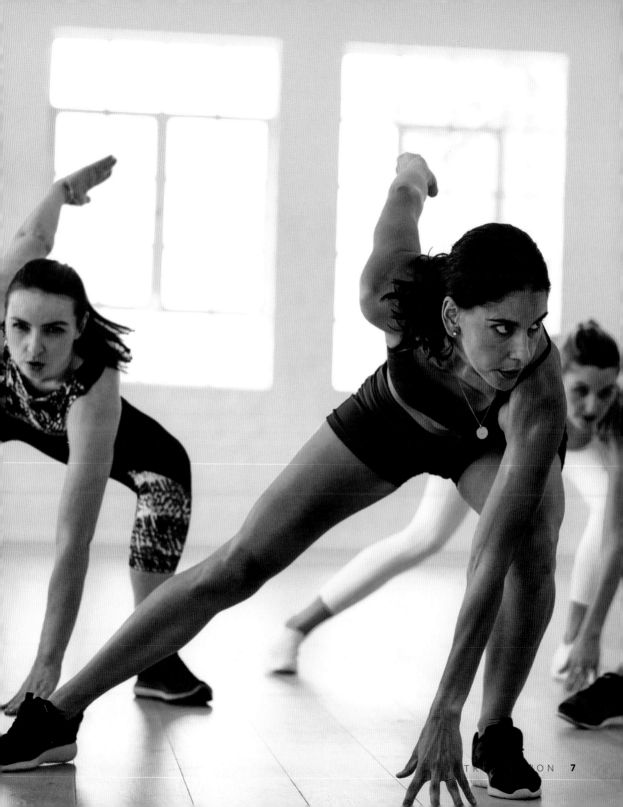

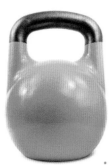

Adding weights to an exercise regime can benefit people of all ages.

Combining your cardio with strength or resistance training is the perfect way to see fast results and make fitness gains in a short period of time. Cardio exercise helps you blitz calories while you are working out, and incorporating interval training (where you work out between different levels) into your cardio workouts will further boost your calorie-burn. Resistance training, or toning exercises, using your body or free/fixed weights to add resistance (for example, a press-up or a bicep curl), will boost your calorie burn after your workout, firstly by creating microtears in the muscles which require energy (calories) to recover and grow. Secondly, resistance work increases your lean muscle mass, which in turn boosts your basal metabolic rate (BMR), meaning your body burns more calories at rest.

Women often don't like to use weights or their bodyweight while working out, but it really is the biggest secret when it comes to toning up, weight-loss and weight maintenance. There's no risk of bulking up as women don't have nearly as much of the hormone testosterone as men, so it's just not possible to achieve the same bulk that men do. To get gorgeous, lean, sculpted muscles, simply try to incorporate weight-training (resistance training) into your routine as often as possible, use low weights (between 2.5 kg (5.5 lb) and 8 kg (17.5 lb)) and aim for higher repetitions, rather than heavier weights and lower reps.

Finally, combine your cardio and strength training exercises with a healthy eating regime and throw in some relaxation techniques and stress-busting yoga moves and you really will be fit for life!

HOW WILL EXERCISE MAKE YOU LOOK AND FEEL YOUNGER?

- **More energy** – doing exercise will give you more energy, meaning you'll be able to go about your normal daily tasks more easily and you'll feel better when you're doing them.

- **Greater mental focus** – it will help to improve mental concentration. Exercise like yoga focuses on developing mental strength, while exercise like running is known to be good for clearing the mind and helping to combat stress.

- **Younger skin** – it will help your skin look younger and more supple. Researchers at McMaster University in Ontario carried out a study on a group of adults aged between 20 and 84. Those who exercised frequently had skin that looked more supple when compared to those who didn't exercise.

- **Better posture** – exercise will help to improve your posture. As your body loses lean muscle tissue and bone density as you get older your posture will change. Weight-bearing exercise like running or strength work can improve bone density, while strength training also helps to increase lean muscle tissue, both of which can prevent your posture from deteriorating.

- **Greater flexibility** – keeping active will help improve your flexibility. This means your muscles and joints won't feel so stiff and you will be able to move more easily.

- **Better sleep** – exercise will help you sleep more easily. Getting good-quality sleep will help you to look and feel younger.

- **Manage your weight** – being regularly active will help you burn calories and keep your weight down, reducing your risk of developing type 2 diabetes or obesity and reducing your risk of heart disease.

- **Slows down the ageing of cells in the body** – telomeres are caps at the end of chromosomes that protect them and therefore slow down ageing. They become shorter with age. Studies have found a link between regular exercise and the length of telomeres, which suggests that doing exercise can slow down the ageing process from the inside out.

You'll sleep more soundly after a workout.

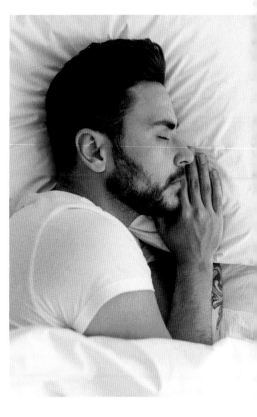

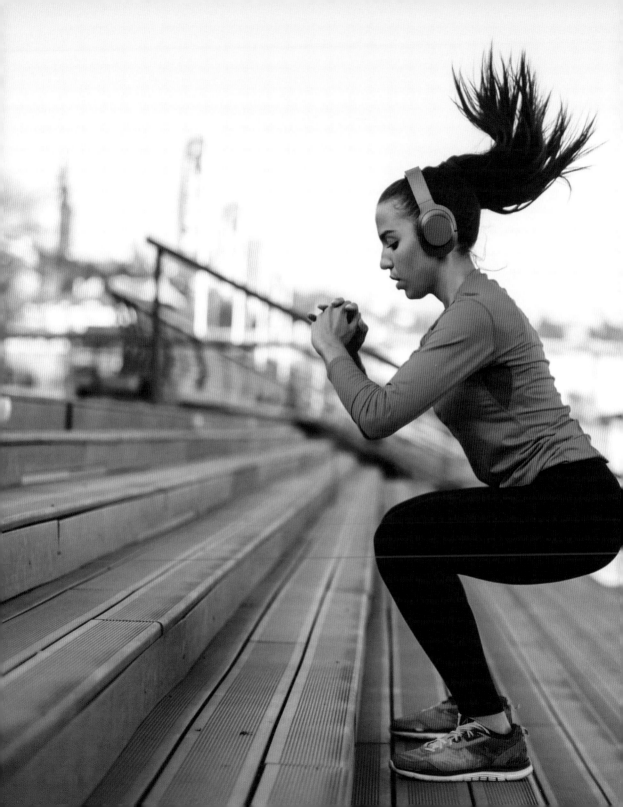

THE IMPORTANCE OF CARDIO

To raise your heart rate and improve your stamina and general fitness, you need to do regular cardiovascular exercise. Walking, running, cycling, swimming, aerobics, rowing, hiking and many kinds of dancing are all 'pure' aerobic activities.

START GETTING FITTER

You can boost your overall fitness, burn more calories and get a leaner, slimmer body with regular cardiovascular exercise. Here's how to get started.

To burn fat and stay lean, you need to include cardiovascular (CV) exercise in your routine at least three to four times per week. If you're new to CV exercise, or you haven't done anything for a while, it's best to start slowly and build up gradually. If you're using the cardio machines in the gym, try to find one you like and one that feels comfortable. The rower and cross-trainer will work the muscles of the upper and lower body, burning more calories because you're working lots of muscle groups. The stationary bike, on the other hand, only works the muscles of the legs. However, a Spin class, where you work hard for intervals of time, will burn a lot of calories – a typical 45-minute class can burn up to 500 calories.

USING THE TREADMILL

The treadmill is also a good option and either running or brisk walking will be effective. If you want to start running but don't think you can run for more than a few minutes, that's OK – just mix running with periods of walking for recovery and build up the running intervals gradually. You might want to run for 30 seconds or one minute, then walk for a minute to recover and then repeat the sequence. As you get fitter, you can decrease the walking intervals and increase the running intervals. Running is an excellent calorie burner, but many people find it challenging at first because they set off too fast. Make sure you jog or run at a comfortable pace. You should be able to maintain a broken conversation and utter a sentence to the person next to you while you're running. Don't try and run like you're sprinting for a bus. There's a reason that sprinters don't run for long – it's extremely hard. Speed doesn't matter so don't worry if your running pace feels or looks slow to begin with. The more often you run the fitter you will get — but make sure you have rest days in between each session. If you're a new runner, you could run on a Monday, Wednesday and Friday, for instance. Give yourself a day of recovery in between the running sessions (you can still do other exercise like yoga or Pilates) so that your muscles can recover. If you want to run outside, use the same interval structure and see how you get on. Time your running intervals or decide you are going to run for the length of a set number of lampposts before you walk to recover. If running isn't your thing, brisk walking with the treadmill on an incline will also burn a lot of calories, as well as engaging your bottom and rear thighs, leading to a firmer, more toned bum and more shapely legs!

REGULAR SESSIONS

Whatever form of cardio exercise you choose, the key is to do it regularly. It's better to do three times a week for 30 minutes each time and keep it up than aim to train every day and skip sessions. A consistent exercise routine will always be more effective than random bursts of a lot of

A treadmill allows you to run or walk whatever the weather. If you have space, you could install one at home but any good gym will have access to the latest models.

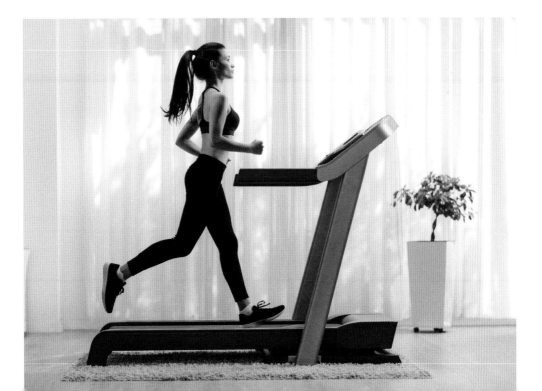

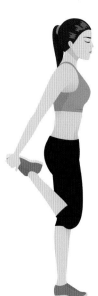

A sequence of stretches will wind down your CV workout effectively.

sessions followed by two weeks of inactivity. Here are some golden rules for getting the most out of your CV sessions:

* Always warm up properly for at least five minutes, either by using the machine of your choice at a low intensity, or another machine that will raise your heart rate. You should feel warm before you start. If you are running outside, begin with a slow walk, picking up into a moderate and then brisk walking pace over a five-minute period.

* Think about your posture when you exercise. If you are running, try to keep your chest up and shoulders high and try to land with your feet under your hips, instead of your feet landing out in front of you (which acts as a braking action and generates more impact through the knees). When doing other CV exercise, stand tall – even if you are sitting on the rower, keep your chest lifted.

* Vary your CV sessions. Fasted cardio, where you exercise first thing in the morning on an empty stomach, can be an effective way to burn more calories, as it will elevate your metabolic rate for the rest of the day. But even introducing more variety into your CV sessions will burn more fat and boost your fitness. Using the random or hill programme on gym machines will work your body harder and boost your results, while doing intervals of working harder followed by periods of more gentle-paced recovery will burn more calories.

* Stretch at the end of every CV session, with particular emphasis on the legs, especially front thighs, rear thighs, bottom and calves. Hold each stretch for at least 30 seconds.

* The body quickly gets used to one type of exercise, so don't be afraid to try a new class in order to shake things up and stimulate your body to work that little bit harder. Good calorie-burning classes include Spin, circuits and Body Attack, Body Combat and Boxercise-style classes.

BEAT THE CLOCK!

You may think that you don't have time to train. But there are many strategies you can use to fit in regular execise.

Q

Why are short workouts effective in terms of fitness and fat burning?

A

Short workouts that are truly HIIT (high-intensity interval training) are proven to improve cardio-respiratory fitness, insulin sensitivity, energy production and fat-free mass. One method, known as the Tabata protocol, is an effective way to burn fat. A full session lasts 20 minutes and can be done on any cardio equipment. Go full intensity for 20 seconds, then take 10 seconds rest, then repeat. Do eight rounds (four minutes), then have a one-minute break and repeat this interval for three more rounds. In total it will take 20 minutes. This is hard, so build up to it! From an exercise scientist's perspective, if you want to optimize fat loss with short workouts, this is currently the most effective way we know.

Q

What's the minimum amount of exercise we can get away with in a workout and still get the benefit?

A

Whatever your fitness level, 30 minutes is all you need to train intensely enough to elevate your heart rate, create a metabolic effect (increased calorie burn) and an elevated after-burn effect (the rate at which you continue to burn calories post-workout). In fact, some research shows 30 minutes to be more effective in improving fitness and weight loss than 60 minutes, as you can typically work a little harder at a high intensity

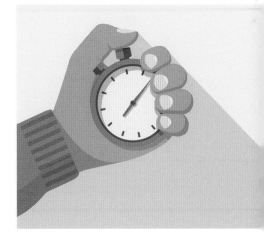

for this shorter duration and therefore keep your heart rate elevated for longer. Shorter workout times lend themselves to more resistance-based exercise, such as weights, resistance bands and circuit training, which builds lean muscle tissue and increases calorie burn.

Q

How do you burn fat and get fit by getting the most out of short workouts?

A

The best workouts for burning fat in a short amount of time are resistance workouts, especially when using HIIT, as it burns lots of calories. For maximum fat loss, do HIIT first thing in the morning in a fasted state (before breakfast). Just 15–20 minutes will put you in a fat-burning zone and you'll continue to burn calories throughout the day. Any type of resistance training will help you burn fat. It doesn't have to be super intense or long. With lower intensity workouts you'll burn fewer calories but they burn a higher percentage of calories from fat than HIIT. For maximum results in a short period of time try planks and all the plank variations (as they work multiple muscles at the same time, most importantly the core), donkey kicks, lying leg kicks, standing leg kicks, clams, glute bridges (as they don't overwork the thighs but focus on the glutes), bear crawls and bicycle crunches. Also handstands against a wall are great for upper body and core strength.

Q

Can short running or cycling sessions still be effective for boosting our fitness?

A

In a word, yes, short runs or cycling sessions can boost fitness levels. According to American College of Sports Medicine guidelines, all adults should participate in up to 150 minutes of moderate activity every week. To simplify, that could work as 30 minutes of activity, five days a week. That's just two per cent of your

30 minutes is all you need to train intensely enough to elevate your heart rate and create a metabolic effect

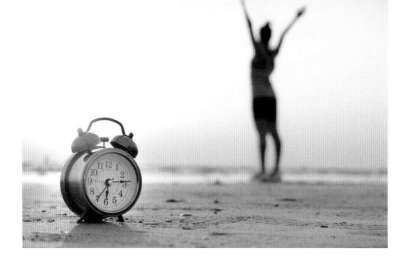

Stake out a time, either daily or on given days in the week and allocate yourself a set time to exercise. You can even time yourself using a stopwatch.

day. To boost your fitness effectively, aim to work at a moderate intensity for a steady state workout – a continuous jog or cycle for 30 minutes, working at 50–70 per cent of your maximum heart rate (HR). Or you can challenge your heart rate by working at 80–90 per cent for 30 seconds before allowing ample recovery, then repeating the interval five to ten times. This is a great way to stimulate different energy systems and avoid overtraining. Using methods like these could reduce your training time to just 20 minutes a session – leaving no excuse not to fit it into your day!

Q
What are the downfalls, if any, of doing shorter workouts?
A
There are no major downfalls for doing shorter workouts unless the type of workout isn't good for your body. Shorter workouts that rely on high intensity usually result in high impact. Recently however, leading trainers have proven you don't need to beat your body up to see results. If you are going to go for HIIT, mix it up with high- and low-impact exercises, such as weight training, functional training and other low-impact styles of training, such as Pilates. You will miss out on some things, like reaching your one-rep max (the maximum amount of weight you can lift in one rep) or drop sets, which take time to move through as they have lots of rest time between sets. However, your heart will still get stronger by doing shorter workouts, so don't worry about that.

WALKING FOR WEIGHT LOSS

You can walk to work, on the beach, in the countryside. Walking barefoot on soft sand gives you something extra to push against, increasing the benefits of your exercise.

Suitable for almost all levels of fitness, walking is completely free, can be fitted in anywhere and if you do it briskly, can give substantial cardiovascular benefits.

Research from the National Walkers' Health Study shows that the further you walk, the more benefits you can reap if you have a condition such as diabetes or high blood pressure. People who completed a walk of 4–6K

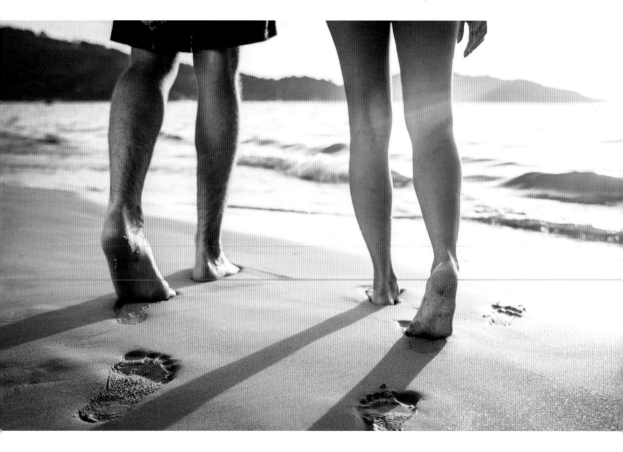

a week had a lower risk of needing anti-diabetic and anti-hypertensive drugs, regardless of how far they walked in total each week. The odds of needing these drugs were around 30 per cent lower in women who had completed a 6–8 km walk each week, compared with those walking less than 4–6 km (2.5–4 miles. Walking can also be an effective way to lose weight if you work at a reasonable intensity. Here's how to get the most out of it.

1 ENGAGE YOUR ARMS

The faster you walk, the more you swing your arms, which helps to increase your speed. A good pace is 4–5.5 miles (6–9 km) an hour. This difference in intensity and effort pays you a big reward, giving you all the weight-loss and toning benefits. As you get fitter, your speed will increase.

2 WALK WHENEVER YOU CAN

As well as your walking workouts, try to build as much walking into your life as possible. Walk to the shops or take a break from work and walk at lunchtime.

3 FIND CHALLENGING TERRAIN

Hilly terrain ups the intensity and gives your legs and butt a great workout. Cross country is another great challenge, as the mixture of terrain means you engage more muscles. Walking on a sandy beach burns around 100 calories per mile. So even while you're on your summer holiday you can stick to your walking plan and keep your mind and body healthy.

4 USE INTERVALS

Introducing bursts of faster walking into your sessions will help to boost your fitness and burn more calories. Aim to walk as fast as you can without breaking into a jog. You could walk fast for one minute, slow down for one minute and repeat. You'll soon get fitter.

CYCLE YOUR WAY
FROM COUCH TO 30K!

You can go faster on a bike. If you cycle to work you can make your commute part of your exercise regime. And a leisure cycle in the country yields similar benefits.

Greener, healthier methods of travel such as cycling are on the increase. The way in which bicycle travel will benefit the environment is clear – more cycling means fewer greenhouse gases – but the boon it might have on public health could be just as great. Cycling provides a low-impact aerobic workout that is great for your heart, brain and blood vessels. It also triggers the release of feel-good endorphins. Cycle to work and you'll be kick-starting your metabolism, burning calories (around 400 calories per hour of gentle cycling), reducing anxiety and improving creative thinking. It's the ideal tonic.

WEEK 1

MONDAY Rest or cross train.
TUESDAY 5–30 minutes at a low intensity. Build bike confidence by changing gears and getting a feel for braking (note which brake controls the front and rear wheels).
WEDNESDAY Rest or cross train.
THURSDAY 30 minutes at a low intensity. Aim for an intensity that enables you to hold a conversation.
FRIDAY Rest.
SATURDAY 30–45 minutes at a low intensity. Aim for around 10 km (6 miles) on a flat route. A hilly route of this distance will take longer.
SUNDAY Rest or cross train.

TOP TIP Set up your bike or let your local bike shop do it. Focus on adjusting the saddle height and making sure you have control of the handlebars and brakes.

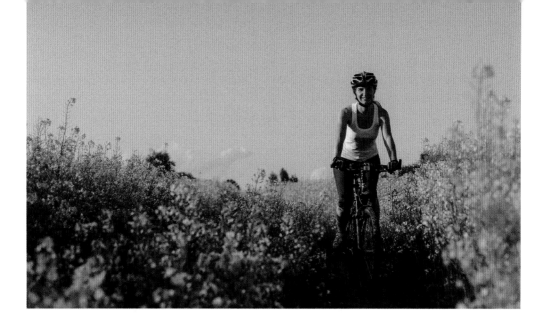

WEEK 2

MONDAY Rest or cross train

TUESDAY 35 minutes at a low intensity. If you feel you can and want to do more, slightly increase the duration rather than pushing yourself harder.

WEDNESDAY Rest or cross train.

THURSDAY 40 minutes at a low intensity. Try and add a little more distance or time to the ride you completed on Tuesday.

FRIDAY Rest.

SATURDAY 45–60 minutes at a low intensity. Aim for 15k+(9–10 miles). If there's a tough hill or traffic roundabout you're not confident enough to manage, pre-plan to walk that section.

SUNDAY Rest or cross train.

TOP TIP Find a quiet stretch of road and practise taking one hand off the handlebars (training for signalling). Focus on keeping pedalling, staying relaxed and looking ahead.

WEEK 3

MONDAY Rest or cross train.

If you like to be outdoors, make the most of your cycle trips to improve your cardiovascular fitness.

TUESDAY 45 minutes, cycled as: 15 mins easy, 2 x (5 mins faster leg speed in same gear, then 5 mins easy), 15 mins easy.

WEDNESDAY Rest or cross train.

THURSDAY 45 minutes, cycled as: 15 mins easy, 2 x (5 mins with an increase of 1–2 gears harder, with slower leg speed, then 5 mins easy), 15 mins easy.

FRIDAY Rest.

SATURDAY 60–80 minutes at a low intensity. Add 5k+ (3 miles) to last week's ride. Practice pedalling speeds and gears on your route, to get a feel for the control you have of the effort. Remember to resort back to easy cycling for the majority of the ride.

SUNDAY Rest or cross train.

TOP TIP Try to maintain a strong core when in a harder gear or higher leg speed – the legs should be doing the work; the upper body shouldn't rock from side to side.

WEEK 4

MONDAY Rest or cross train.

TUESDAY 55 minutes, cycled as: 15 mins easy, 3 x (5 mins faster leg speed same gear, then 5 mins easy), 15 mins easy.

WEDNESDAY

Rest or cross train.

THURSDAY 55 minutes, cycled as: 15 mins easy, 3 x (5 mins with an increase of 1–2 gears harder, with lower leg speed, then 5 mins easy), 15 mins easy.

FRIDAY Rest.

SATURDAY 90 minutes+ at a low intensity. You're ready to complete your 30k (19 mile) ride if you wish to do so! Take your time and enjoy it.

SUNDAY Rest or cross train.

TOP TIP It's wise to practice your full commute at least once during this week, so you know the roads, the junctions and time it takes you to commute in.

STEP UP!

Never mind the latest fancy fitness fads. Climbing the stairs – in the home and outdoors – is an easy, accessible and budget-friendly way to burn calories, reduce blood pressure and even lower your brain age.

You don't need an expensive gym membership or even a decent pair of trainers to get fit. It turns out that the perfect tool for total body and mind health was staring us in the face the whole time (or rather, 'stairing'). Climbing the stairs at home, work or out and about is one of the simplest, most effective ways to give your heart, brain and muscles a boost. Here's why.

A WAY TO WEIGHT LOSS

Stair climbing burns 8–11 calories per minute and adding in two flights daily can lead to 6 lbs (2.7 km) of weight loss over just one year, according to a US study. And no wonder– it's twice as taxing as a brisk walk, according to Harvard research, and 50 per cent more challenging than walking up a steep incline. 'Stair climbing is a great calorie burner. It's

Take the stairs wherever you are to boost your fitness. Whether it's climbing an escalator rather than letting it carry you or jogging up flights of outdoor steps, all are beneficial.

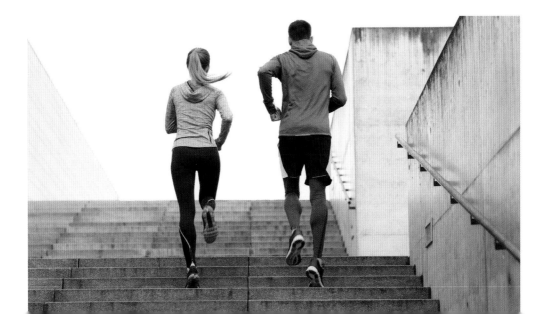

a combination of cardio and strength training which will tone and build stamina,' says personal trainer Becks Boston. 'Add ankle weights increase the effort and hold a pair of light dumbbells for extra resistance and this will improve your core stability which will tone your stomach muscles and help your posture.'

IMPROVED HEART HEALTH

Another reason to step up – researchers from Canada revealed that stair climbing increases cardiovascular fitness. The even better news is that, while previous studies have found similar results based on prolonged stair climbing, this research found short, sharp bursts could yield similar results. Participants climbed vigorously up and down one flight for 60 seconds, totalling 30 minutes a week – an exercise that's really easy to replicate at home or work. This heart health benefit could be why stair climbing has been linked with living a longer life. The Harvard Alumni Study found that men who climb eight flights of stairs a day on average have a 33 per cent lower mortality rate than men who are inactive – even higher than those who walk 1.3 miles a day. While Step Aerobics used to be all the rage, it's less common to find classes at the gym. Luckily YouTube has stepped in – you'll find lots of free step sessions including some made by Reebok that will get your heart pumping.

MAGIC FOR MENOPAUSE

Going through menopause can cause a reduction in your muscle strength as oestrogen levels decrease. But researchers from the North American Menopause Society discovered that stair climbing is great for building leg strength – especially in post-menopausal women. The same research also demonstrated it can lower blood pressure and reduce your risk of osteoporosis. Participants trained for four days a week climbing 192 steps between two and five times each day.

RAISE YOUR ENERGY

When flagging, you might be tempted to reach for a caffeinated drink, but there's a simple, natural alternative. Yes, you guessed it – going up and down the stairs! Just 10 minutes of this was found to make people feel more energized than drinking 50 milligrams of coffee, according to an American study. The remedy is now being recommended for sluggish office workers. For more motivation to take the stairs at work, it's worth knowing that stair climbing can be built up through the course of the day, making a significant contribution to your daily physical activity. It is good for the heart, muscle strength and bone density.

GOOD FOR YOUR BRAIN

While getting your steps in is obviously good for your body, there's evidence it's also great for your grey matter. In fact, the more stairs you climb, the younger your brain appears to get, according to a Canadian study. Researchers found that people's brain age decreased by 0.58 years for every daily flight of stairs they climbed. This was found by measuring their grey matter through MRI scanners.

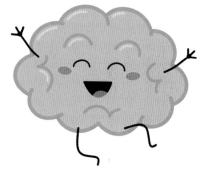

IT'S NOT ALL ABOUT GOING UP …

Walking back down the stairs has its own set of unique benefits. It's a form of eccentric exercise, which means placing a load on a muscle when it's lengthening, rather than shortening (as happens on the way up). Going downstairs was found to reduce the risk of diabetes in a group of obese women in an Australian study, lowering their resting levels of insulin and glucose as well as increasing their levels of good cholesterol. Need motivation? Sign up for a Tower Run (towerrunninguk.com), a bit like a normal race but – you guessed it – climbing a tower or landmark.

GET YOUR STEPS

When you aim for a certain number of stairs a day, you'll start seeing them everywhere! Avoid escalators and lifts in shops and stations and use the toilets or coffee machine on different floors of your workplace. Make a day trip of it – Southwold Lighthouse in Suffolk has 113 steps, St Paul's Cathedral in London has 528, and Blackpool Tower has a whopping 1,036!

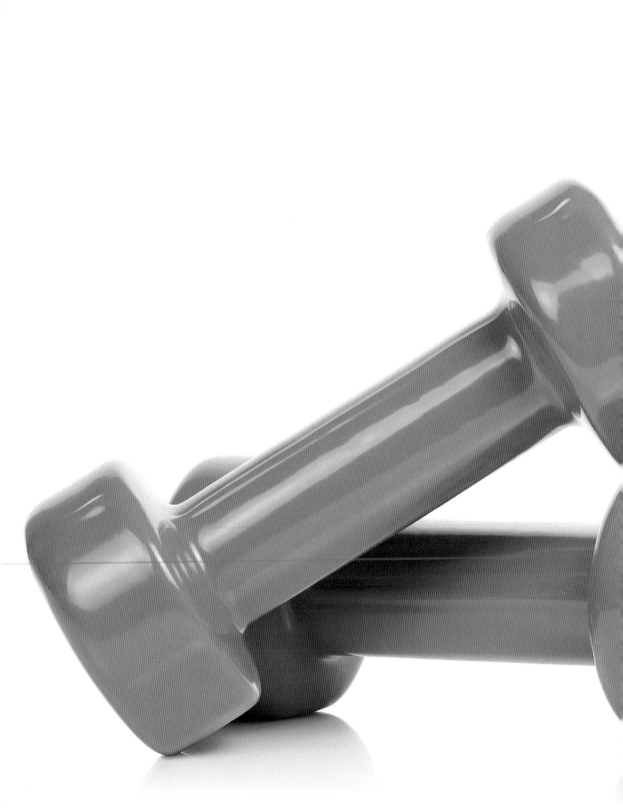

WHY YOU NEED STRENGTH TRAINING

The importance of strength training cannot be overstated whatever your age or fitness level. It strengthens your bones and helps to build leaner, more efficient muscles.

SHAPE UP, FEEL STRONGER AND LEANER!

Strength training will give you a firmer, leaner body and help you look and feel younger. It will also reduce your risk of osteoporosis. Here's how to get started.

Call it what you will: strength training, weight training, resistance training. The name doesn't matter. Just make sure you include some regular strength training in your weekly exercise schedule. When you lift weights, your muscle tone improves, so you have a firmer, more shapely body. You'll also reap numerous health benefits that will result in you looking and feeling younger. Here's why you should include strength training in your workouts:

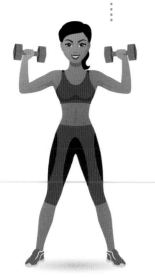

BURN MORE FAT

From the age of about 30, our bodies begin to lose muscle mass. Weight training enables us to build lean muscle tissue, which is more metabolically active, meaning your body will not only burn calories during exercise, but also at rest.

IMPROVED BONE DENSITY

It will reduce your risk of osteoporosis, which currently affects one in two women in the UK over the age of 50. Studies have shown that if women were to participate in weight training for just 20 minutes, four times a week for ten years before the onset of the menopause, osteoporosis would be unlikely to occur in later life. Incidentally, peak bone density is reached by around 25 to 35 years of age. After that, we lose about one per cent of bone density per year.

From the age of about 30, our bodies begin to lose muscle mass

GREATER QUALITY OF LIFE

As you get stronger, daily tasks that involve lifting or carrying objects will begin to feel easier.

STRENGTHEN MORE THAN JUST MUSCLES

Strength training doesn't just make your muscles stronger, it also strengthens your tendons and ligaments, which will help your body function well. Also, strong muscles act as shock absorbers for joints. The stronger they are, the more they can absorb shock.

BETTER BODY ALIGNMENT

Muscle imbalances can be overcome to correct your posture, and weak muscles can be targeted with strength training to overcome a muscle imbalance. For instance, if you have strong quadriceps (front thighs) but weak hamstrings (rear thighs), you should focus more on exercises for hamstrings.

You don't need to use weights to do strength training. Exercises that use your bodyweight such as push-ups are highly effective.

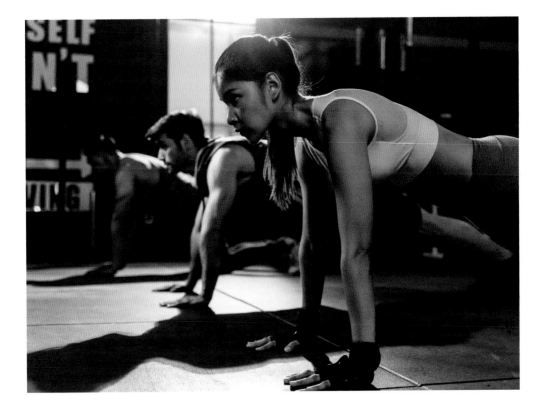

HOW TO USE WEIGHTS

ALWAYS ASK A GYM INSTRUCTOR to show you safe technique. If you're new to resistance training, using machines like Leg Press (opposite, top), Lat Pull Down (for upper back – opposite below), Chest Press and Shoulder Press is a good way to start as these machines all move in a fixed plane of movement.

- Start with two sets of 12–15 repetitions, then add another set after four to six weeks.

- Use a slow and controlled technique – don't use momentum to help you.

- Work large muscle groups first, like legs and back, then work smaller muscles like chest, shoulders and triceps (rear upper arms).

- When doing standing exercises like squats and lunges, be aware of your posture. Keep your chest lifted when squatting and keep your upper body upright when doing lunges.

- Have a rest period of 30 seconds to one minute in between each set.

- Leave core exercises like the plank until the end, as you will want your core muscles to engage and support you when you are lifting weights. They are less likely to be able to do this if you train them first and they are fatigued.

- Stretch at the end of each exercise to avoid post-exercise soreness (if you're new to weights you may still feel a little bit sore the next day). Hold each stretch for at least 30 seconds.

- Rest in between sessions – never train the same muscle group two days in a row. Muscles typically take up to 48 hours to recover in between strength-training sessions.

- If you intend to use weights three to four times a week, try a split routine where, for instance, you work lower-body muscles one day and upper body the next.

- Increase the weight if the exercise begins to feel easy. The last two or three reps of a set should feel challenging. If you complete 15 reps knowing that you could easily have performed another five then the weight is too light.

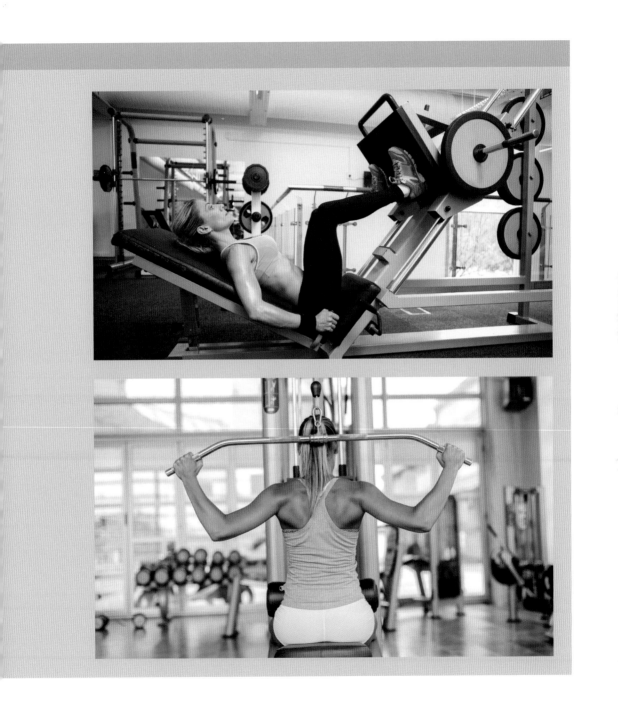

TRIM AND TONED

Strength exercises can significantly improve the shape and tone of your body, creating a firmer, more sculpted figure.

RESISTANCE BAND TRICEPS PRESS-DOWN
AREA TRAINED: Rear upper arms

TECHNIQUE: Tie a resistance band around a secure object slightly higher than your head. Hold the edges in your hands with your arms bent. Keep your elbows tucked into your sides. Push your hands down towards your legs. Slowly return with control. Perform two sets of 15 to 20 repetitions.

Be safe

Ensure that you always have tension in the resistance band.

RESISTANCE BAND SEATED ROW
AREA TRAINED: Upper back

TECHNIQUE: Sit on the floor with your back and legs straight. Place a resistance band around both feet. Grab hold of the edges of the resistance band. Pull your elbows backwards, squeezing your shoulder blades together. Slowly return to the starting position. Perform two sets of 15 to 20 repetitions.

Be safe

Don't slouch when doing this exercise.

RESISTANCE BAND CRAB WALK
AREA TRAINED: Bottom

TECHNIQUE: Stand with both feet together on a resistance band. Cross the resistance band in front of your body and hold the edges in your hands. Ensure that you have a medium amount of tension in the band. Keep your back straight. Take five steps to one side and five steps back. Perform two sets of 15 to 20 repetitions.

Be safe

Keep your stomach muscles tight and look straight ahead.

RESISTANCE BAND TORSO TWIST

AREAS TRAINED: Back, sides, stomach, core

TECHNIQUE: Tie a resistance band around a secure object about chest height. Stand with your side facing the resistance band. Twist your body slightly towards the resistance band. Hold the edges with both hands. Keep your arms straight. Rotate your body to the opposite side pulling on the resistance band. Slowly release the tension and return to the starting position. Complete one set before changing over to the other side. Perform two sets of 15 to 20 repetitions on both sides.

Be safe

Keep your core muscles contracted and perform slow, controlled movements.

CHEST FLY

AREA TRAINED: Chest

TECHNIQUE: Lie on your back on a step or an exercise ball. Hold a weight in each hand with your palms facing each other. Keep a slight bend in your elbows. Open your arms sideways and lower the weights until they are almost level with your shoulders. Slowly bring your arms back up to the starting position. Perform two sets of 15 to 20 repetitions.

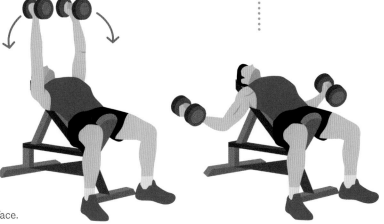

Be safe

Always keep the weights over your chest, not your face.

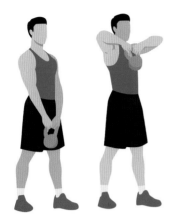

UPRIGHT ROW
AREAS TRAINED: Upper back and neck
TECHNIQUE: Stand upright and hold a weight with both hands in front of your body. Pull the weight up to your chin, lifting your elbows higher than your shoulders. Slowly lower with control. Perform two sets of 15 to 20 repetitions.

Be safe
Keep your back straight and your core muscles contracted.

CRISS CROSS
AREAS TRAINED: Stomach and side muscles
TECHNIQUE: Lie on your back on the floor with your knees bent at a right angle and your hands next to your head. Tuck your tailbone in and pull your belly button in towards your spine. Inhale. Crunch up with your shoulders, rotating your shoulder towards the opposite knee while extending the other leg to a 45-degree angle. Exhale. Return to the centre position and repeat to the other side. Perform two sets of 15 repetitions on each side.

Be safe
Ensure that your lower back doesn't arch off the floor.

SUPERMAN
AREAS TRAINED: Upper back, deeper back muscles
TECHNIQUE: Lie down on your stomach on the floor with your arms extended above your head. Lift one arm and the opposite leg. Inhale. Hold the position for two breaths. Exhale while lowering with control and repeat on the other side. Perform two sets of 15 repetitions on each side.

Be safe
Don't roll your hips when lifting your legs.

HUNDREDS
AREA TRAINED: Stomach
TECHNIQUE: Lie on your back on the floor with your knees at right angles and your arms next to your body, palms down. Inhale. Exhale, crunching your shoulders off the floor and keeping your chin tucked in, reaching through your fingertips. Keep your shoulders down. Stay in this position while you inhale. Pumping up and down with your arms, breathe in for five beats, out for five beats, and so on. After 100 beats bend your knees and curl back down.

Be safe
Ensure that your back stays in contact with the floor.

INCLINE STRAIGHT-ARMSIDE-STAR PLANK
AREAS TRAINED: Shoulder, side muscles, stomach
TECHNIQUE: Place one hand on a step directly underneath your shoulder and the other arm extended up to the ceiling. Inhale. Keep your body and legs in a straight line in a side plank position. Keep your core muscles tight. Exhale. Lift your top leg up to form a star shape. Hold for 15 to 30 seconds before changing over to the other side. Focus on slow, controlled breathing.

Be safe
If you find the exercise too hard, perform the side plank without lifting your leg.

BRIDGE TO CRUNCHES
AREAS TRAINED: Back muscles, bottom, rear thighs, stomach muscles, core
TECHNIQUE: Lie on your back, keeping your knees bent and feet firmly on the floor. Inhale. Squeeze a towel or pillow in between your knees.

Contract your core muscles and curl your tailbone off the floor. Exhale. Lift your spine vertebra by vertebra off the floor. Inhale. Slowly lower with control, placing your back down bone by bone. Exhale. Relax your tailbone. Inhale. Curl your upper body off the floor, keeping your chin tucked in. Exhale. Reach with your fingertips towards your ankles. Lower your upper body. Inhale. Perform two sets of five to eight repetitions.

Be safe

Perform slow, controlled movements to improve mobility in your spine.

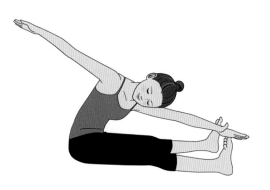

SAW

AREAS TRAINED: Back, side muscles, inner thighs, back thighs

TECHNIQUE: Sit on the floor with your legs a comfortable distance apart and extend your arms to the sides. Inhale, lengthen your spine and rotate to one side. Exhale and extend the opposite arm to the outside of the opposite leg's little toe. Your other arm is straight reaching up behind you. Hold the position for two breaths. Exhale, lengthen your spine and rotate back to the centre. Alternate between each side. Perform two sets of ten repetitions on each side.

Be safe

Don't force your knees down if you don't have the flexibility. Keep them slightly bent.

LEG PULL-IN

AREAS TRAINED: Shoulders, hips, rear thighs, stomach muscles

TECHNIQUE: Start with your hands by your sides with your arms slightly bent at the elbow and your legs out in front of you. Bend your knees and using your abdominals, draw them in towards your chest, ensuring that your feet stay together. Exhale.

Slowly extend your legs to return to the starting position. Repeat for five to ten repetitions.

Be safe

Ensure that you don't drop your hips when you kick your leg up.

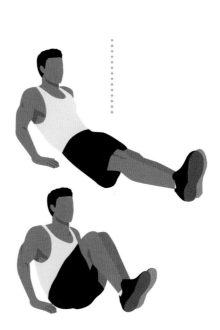

DART INTO SIDE BEND
AREAS TRAINED: Back muscles, side muscles

TECHNIQUE: Lie on your stomach on the floor — squeeze your inner thighs to bring them together and hold it throughout the movement. Inhale. Contract your core, rotate your palms in to face your thighs and reach your fingertips towards your feet. Your head will lift up. Exhale. Hold this position for one breath. Bend sideways from the waist, gliding your arm down your leg. Exhale. Hold this position for one breath. Return to the centre position and repeat on the other side. Perform two sets of eight to ten repetitions on each side.

Be safe

Don't lift up too high and ensure that you keep your head aligned with your spine.

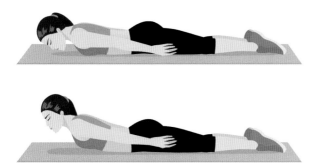

IN PEAK CONDITION

If you're stuck in a rut it's easy to get super fit and strong with these key moves for those who want to work hard and challenge their body for best results.

TWIST JUMPS

Good for raising your heart rate

- Stand with your feet hip-width apart and your arms at a right angle at your sides.
- Keep your knees slightly bent.
- Twist your upper body towards the right.
- Jump up.
- Twist your legs over to the right and your upper body over to the left.
- Land allowing your knees to bend to absorb the shock.
- Alternate as fast as possible for a minute.

Tip: Keep your back upright and focus on one point in front of you, rather than twisting your head with the movement.

BACKWARD LUNGES WITH OVERHEAD RAISES (RIGHT)

Good for your legs, shoulders and cardiovascular fitness

- Stand with your legs hip-width apart.
- Hold a weight with both hands in front of your body.
- Step backwards with your left leg and bend both knees to lunge.
- While lunging, lift the weight with both arms over your head.
- Step forwards to the start position.
- Repeat with your right leg.
- Alternate between left and right.

Tip: Keep your upper body upright – don't lean forward.

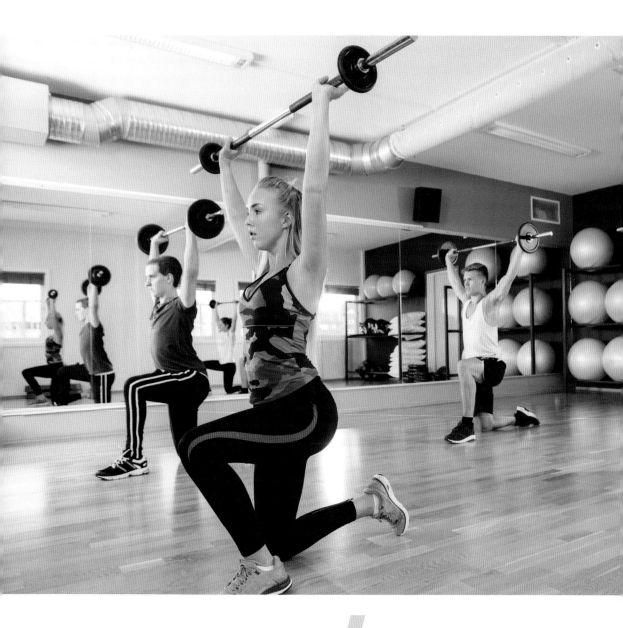

When lunging, always keep your
upper body upright

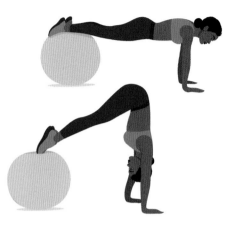

STABILITY BALL PIKES

Good for your core and upper body

- Place your feet on a stability ball.
- Place your hands on the floor.
- Keep a straight line between your shoulders, hips and feet.
- Roll the ball closer to your hands while pushing your bottom up to the ceiling.
- Roll the ball back to the starting position.

Tip: Perform the move slowly.

KNEELING STABILITY BALL ROLL OUTS

Good for your core

- Kneel on the floor behind a stability ball.
- Place your elbows and forearms on the ball.
- Lean forward with your hips to form a straight line between your knees, hips and shoulders.
- Push your arms forward and roll the ball out.
- Pull your arms back in until your elbows are underneath your shoulders.
- Keep your hips in the same position throughout the movement.

Tip: To make the exercise easier, perform it with your knees on the floor.

RESISTANCE BAND CRUNCHES

Good for your abs

- Tie a resistance band around a secure object.
- Lie on your back on the floor.
- Hold the ends of the resistance band in your hands and keep your hands next to your ears.
- Ensure that there is slight tension in the band.
- Crunch your head and shoulders up off the floor, pulling on the resistance band.
- Slowly lower with control.

Tip: Support your neck with your hands if it hurts. Breathe out as you crunch up.

DOUBLE LEG STRETCHES

Good for your core and abs

- Lie on your back on the floor and keep your legs at a right angle, with your shins parallel to the floor.
- Crunch your head and shoulders off the floor.
- Tuck your knees into your abs and push your lower back into the floor.
- Grab hold of your shins with your hands.
- Breathe out.
- Stretch your arms above your head and stretch your legs out to a 45-degree angle.
- Keep your head off the floor and your lower back into the floor.
- Breathe out.
- Take your arms sideways into a semi-circle and tuck your knees in again, grabbing hold of your shins.
- Repeat the move.

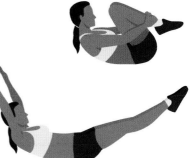

Tip: The closer your arms are to the floor, the harder it is to stop your back from arching.

LUNGES TO SINGLE LEG STANCES

Good for legs and glutes

- Stand with your feet hip-width apart.
- Lunge forward with your left leg and bend both knees.
- As you lift up, push off with your left leg into a single leg balancing stance on your right leg.
- Perform 12 repetitions each side.

Tip: Keep your upper back upright.

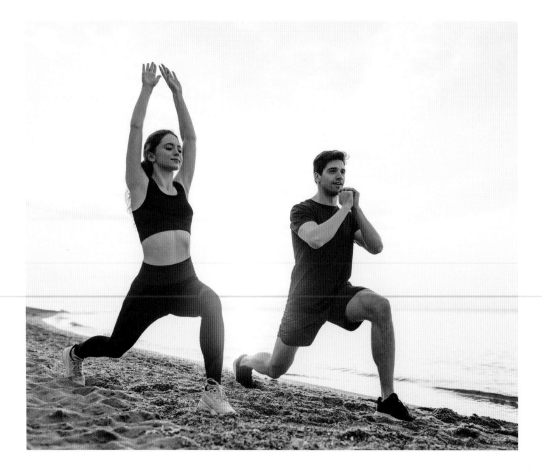

TWO BEST AB MOVES

PUSHED FOR TIME? If you only do two ab exercises, these two moves will bring great results.

1. Straight arm and leg crunches
Good for the mid-section

- Lie on your back, extend your right arm above your head and extend your right leg.
- Place your left hand behind your head and keep your left leg at a right angle.
- Crunch your right arm and leg up until your hand touches your leg.
- Slowly return to the starting position.
- Perform one set on one side, then change over (try two to three sets of 12–15 repetitions).

Tip: Tilt your pelvis and breathe out as you lift.

2. Cycling
Good for the mid-section and lower abs. Try to perform this exercise for up to one minute without stopping

- Lie on your back and bend your legs, so you form a right angle at your knees.
- Keep your hands next to your ears.
- Crunch your left elbow over to your right knee while extending your left leg.
- Return to the centre position.
- Crunch your right elbow over to your left knee while extending your right leg.
- Alternate between right and left.

Tip: Keep the tempo controlled.

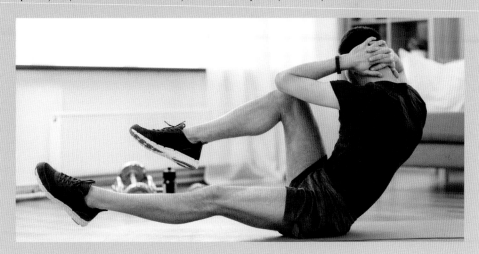

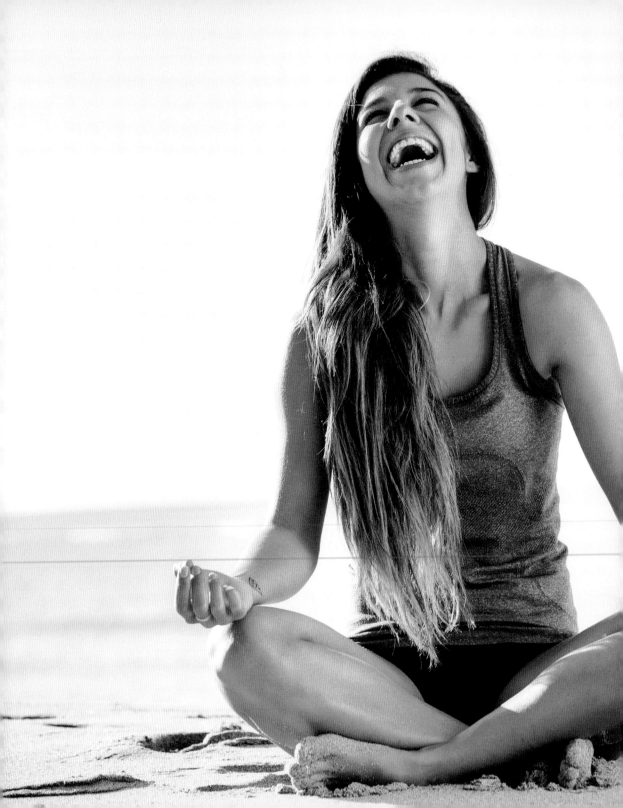

A HEALTHIER LIFESTYLE

It's not just about exercise. How you deal with stress, what you eat and making sure you have enough 'me' time will all contribute to a more healthy way of life.

FIVE-MINUTE STRESS-BUSTERS!

Don't let stress ruin your day – try our simple techniques to soothe frazzled nerves in a matter of minutes!

Life can be hectic sometimes! From heavy workloads and office deadlines to school runs and busy household schedules, we're juggling so many balls it's no wonder we feel the pressure sometimes. But what happens when it all gets on top of you? 'While it is natural to feel anxiety occasionally, it can impact negatively on your life if you feel it constantly or especially strongly,' says Dr Aaron Balick, clinical psychotherapist and author of *The Little Book of Calm*. 'The good news is that you don't need to be powerless in the face of your anxiety. You can learn to control it, and some of the ways to do that are actually quite simple.' Here are a few of our favourites:

HAVE A CUPPA!

All those old wives' tales were right – a soothing brew really does work wonders! Researchers at the University College of London found that people who drank black tea were able to de-stress more quickly than those who drank a fake tea substitute.

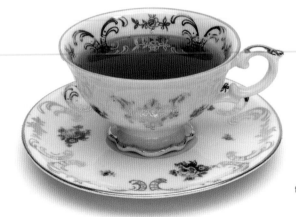

TRY THE 4-7-8 METHOD

This is a brilliant technique derived from yogic breathing to melt tension away. Just place the tip of your tongue on the roof of your mouth behind your teeth, breathe in through your nose for a count of four, hold it for seven then blow air out forcefully through your mouth for a count of eight. Repeat this two or three times whenever you feel stressed or anxious.

RUB YOUR EARS

According to the ancient Chinese art of
acupressure, pressing gently on certain points of
your body can unblock energy and bring about
healing on many levels. Giving yourself a gentle
ear massage activates some of the best pressure
points for instant relaxation. Just gently massage
your ears with your thumb and forefinger, pull
down gently on the lobes and rub the inner
surface of the ear for two to three minutes.

BLOW UP A BALLOON

This is a brilliant tension-buster as it makes you
breathe deeply and slowly into your diaphragm
— a bit like a breathing meditation. When you're
stressed, you tend to take short, shallow breaths,
which starves your body of oxygen. Taking the
deep breaths to blow up a balloon activates your
parasympathetic nervous system, which reduces
your heart rate and relaxes your muscles.

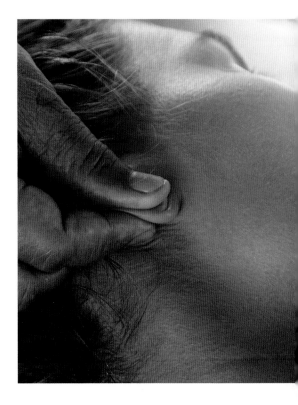

WORK UP A SWEAT

Exercise is a great way to beat anxiety as it helps to release those
fabulous feel-good hormones. And while you might not feel like hitting
the gym after a long day at work it actually helps you to increase your
long-term energy levels, making you feel like you can accomplish
anything!

LAUGH OUT LOUD

Research shows that children laugh an average of 140 times a day while
us miserable adults only manage a paltry 12 to 14 times. 'There's a lot
to be said about laughing,' says psychotherapist Robert Friedman. 'You
release an endorphin every time you laugh, and those are 200 times
stronger than morphine.'

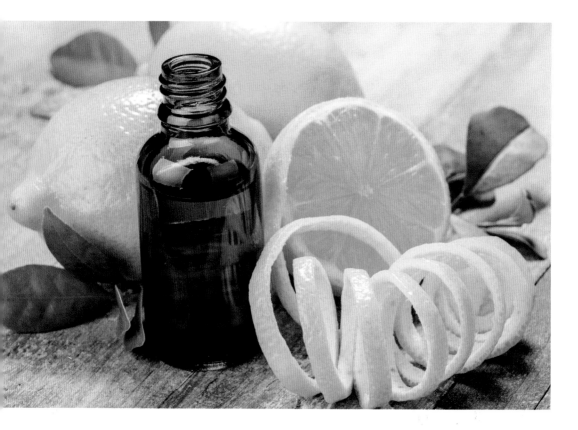

SNIFF A LEMON

Aromatherapy is renowned for its ability to combat stress and now Japanese researchers have found that linalool, a substance found in lemons, may turn down the classic 'flight-or-fight' stress response. Can't find any lemons? Essential oils of lavender, rose, jasmine, clary sage and bergamot are also great soothing scents.

PRACTISE MINDFULNESS

Paying attention to the present is a great way to calm anxiety, says Dr Balick. 'Try this mindfulness technique, which is like a walking meditation. You can do it almost anywhere, indoors or out – just make sure it's quiet and you won't be interrupted.' Just like a sitting meditation, set yourself a time (ten minutes to start should do) during which you walk mindfully for just ten to fifteen paces. Stop. Breathe. And when you're ready, walk back, and stop to breathe again on the other side. While you're walking mindfully notice your natural breathing, the weight of your feet on the ground, the way your body moves. If your thoughts wander, gently bring them back to your walk or your breath.

CLEVER COLOURS

Surrounding yourself with soothing greens or blues is a great way to soothe frazzled nerves as different colours produce different emotional and physical effects. A US study found that red environments increase stress responses, while green and blue environments keep you calm.

STRIKE A POSE

Yoga is a fantastic way to chill your bones as it lowers blood pressure and reduces tension held in the body. Try this simple exercise known as the child's pose. Kneel on the floor on all fours then sit your bottom back on to your heels and stretch your arms forward, lowering your head to the floor. Let your entire body release, feel the tension flooding out of you and hold for a couple of minutes, or for as long as you like! See Chapter Five (page 112) for more soothing yoga poses.

STRESS-BUSTING SNACKS

MUNCH ON THESE TASTY TREATS to soothe away tension

Turkey – contains an amino acid called L-tryptophan that triggers the release of the feel-good brain chemical serotonin

Avocados – rich in stress-relieving B vitamins
and potassium, which helps to lower blood pressure

Salmon – a great source of omega-3 fatty acids, which lower levels of stress hormones such as cortisol and adrenaline

Asparagus – one of the best sources of mood-boosting folic acid

Chocolate – contains phenylethylamine, which encourages your brain to release feel-good endorphins that relax your mind and body.

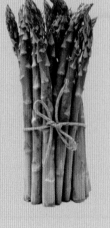

THE GREAT OUTDOORS

Embrace the great outdoors and benefit from what the Scandinavians call 'friluftsliv' for top-to-toe wellbeing

When it comes to understanding the healing effects of nature, no one does al fresco living quite like the Scandinavians. And they have a word for it – 'friluftsliv' (pronounced free-loofts-liv), which translates as 'open-air living'. What's more, it's known to decrease anxiety and depression. With 70 per cent of the world's population predicted to live in an urban setting by 2050, the need to reconnect with nature to stay healthy in body and mind is more important than ever. Friluftsliv is a concept that's ingrained in the Nordic way of life from childhood onwards. 'Put simply, it means doing something outdoors. This could be walking in the forest with a picnic, enjoying a small fika (coffee and cake) break in the open air or doing something more organised such as walking in the mountains,' says Lena Köpcke, chief of people and culture at Fishbrain (fishbrain.com), an app that encourages people to embrace the great outdoors.

From waterside feasts to weekend hikes, it turns out a typical Scandi day is just as idyllic as we'd imagine, combining socialising and outdoor activities – all without a smartphone in sight. 'I wake up, make a packed lunch and put it into a backpack, along with any other essentials, then either cycle or take a walk to a beautiful outdoor space with friends or family,' says Lena. 'In the summer, we will pick berries or mushrooms in the forest, rent a kayak or paddleboard and spend the day on the water, or in the winter, we do the same thing, but we ski or skate on the ice.'

Despite living in often sub-zero temperatures Scandinavians have a genuine love of al fresco living and are better off for it – after all, the region is often dubbed one of the happiest places in the world. 'Our bodies are made to move and we need the sun and fresh air to function,' says Lena. 'In Sweden, people typically live near large nature spots so it has become part of our culture to spend time outside.' Even though we may not have acres of Nordic forests here in the UK, we've still got some pretty amazing

Getting outside with children means you can play and run while also getting the benefit of fresh air and peaceful space.

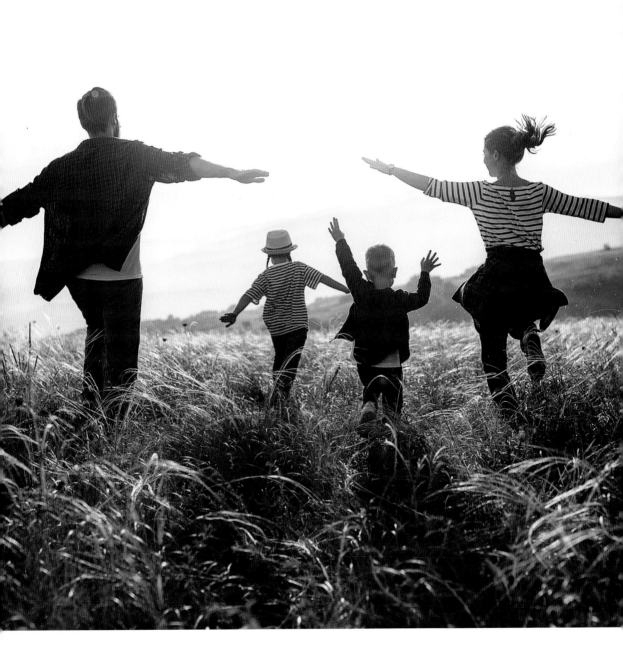

countryside in which to roam. 'Just make sure whatever you do doesn't feel like a chore or a fitness "must-do," and that it's for pure enjoyment – that's what's at the heart of friluftsliv', says Lena. So why not make the most of our countryside? You'll be doing your body and mind the world of good.

ALL GOOD IN THE WOOD

No mountains or even hills near you? Try seeking out local woodland instead. A study has linked being among trees to lower stress levels, reduced depression and better sleep. The recent study, led by Professor Richard Mitchell at Glasgow University, revealed a 50 per cent improvement in people's mental health if they were physically active in a natural environment. One of the reasons for this lies with tiny particles called phytoncides – airborne particles with antibacterial and antifungal qualities emitted by leafy plants. The plants produce them to protect themselves from insects, but it turns out they're beneficial to human health too!

Strolling through soft sand or splashing through the shallows is great for positive energy.

WATER WONDERS

Walking on a beach listening to the waves is a great way to get a health fix. A study by the University of Exeter found that the rhythmic sound of ocean waves has a positive effect on your brain, which in turn encourages a more peaceful pace of thought. And it's not just the sound that soothes. 'Sea air is charged with negative ions, which helps boost oxygen levels in your blood and makes you feel more energised,' says Chris Naylor, author of *Go Wild: Find Freedom and Adventure in the Great Outdoors.* 'The salt in the water vapour also has a positive effect on natural mood-boosters tryptamine, serotonin, and melatonin, which can lead to a better night's sleep.'

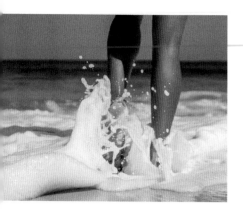

CLIMB EVERY MOUNTAIN

While tackling steep, rocky terrain may not be a daily occurrence for you, heading up to higher ground now and then could do wonders for your physical health. A report published in the *Journal of Epidemiology and Community Health* found that people who spent time at higher altitudes reduced their risk of heart disease. This is because the altitude reduces oxygen, which causes your body to create new blood vessel pathways, allowing for greater oxygen flow. Plus, being free from pollutants and toxins, the high mountain air is good for you in other ways: it has been proven to strengthen your immune system, boost metabolism and even reduce respiratory problems, such as asthma.

EMBRACE THE OUTDOORS

- PUT YOUR BEST FOOT FORWARD Walking is the perfect way to embrace friluftsliv. 'Find time each day to walk for the sake of walking. Go for a stroll during your lunch break or have a walk before or after work to get moving and breathing the fresh air,' says Chris.

- OBSERVE THE BIRDS Birds are everywhere – even in urban environments. Becoming a twitcher is a meditative activity that requires patience and mental alertness, but allows you a little time for peace and quiet without modern distractions. Visit the RSPB's website (rspb.org.uk) where you can learn how to identify our feathered friends.

- FORGO THE CAR Cycling to work allows you to spend more time in the open air. And it's all part of the friluftsliv life – around 50 per cent of Copenhagen residents commute to work by bike and another 25 per cent of them walk.

- PACK UP A PICNIC Whatever the weather, gathering with others for a meal outdoors is an integral part of Scandi life. Not only has eating outdoors been shown by scientists to improve your concentration and memory, but breaking bread with others is a great opportunity to stop, listen and be listened to, and develop invaluable empathy skills.

- ADD GREENERY TO YOUR LIVING SPACE You needn't be a gardening guru to reap the rewards of nature. Indoor plants boost your wellbeing by reducing levels of carbon dioxide, benzene, nitrogen dioxide and even dust. 'Whether it's a tiny succulent or a big and beautiful cheese plant, greenery at home or work provides an easy way to bring nature into your everyday,' says Chris.

SHAKE IT OFF

Could making your muscles quiver help release tension from your life?

Do a quick scan of your body now – are you clenching your jaw? Are your shoulders tensed up around your ears? If you carry stress in your tightened muscles without really noticing, you're not alone. But help could be at hand from an unlikely source – giving yourself a good shake. Trauma Release Exercises (TRE) are simple movements designed to let your body shake, which is believed to release tension, stress and trauma. Developed in the 1990s by Dr David Berceli, it's been used around the world to help release people from anything from day-to-day anxieties, to the symptoms of PTSD in war zones. 'Our stress response is designed to help us escape an enemy, such as a tiger,' says Steve Haines, the UK's leading TRE practitioner. 'Your muscles get tight, your heart starts pumping and your pupils get wider.

'Obviously there are certain circumstances where that's useful, but many people find that the pressures of modern life leave this response "switched on", which can overload your heart, make you tired and cause anxiety. It also means that your body doesn't prioritise non-urgent systems such as digestion or your immune system. This kind of stress is implicated in just about every health problem you can suffer.' Left unchecked, stress can cause issues with libido, fertility and digestive problems and, of course, make you feel very unhappy. Chronic stress has been shown to affect the body's inflammatory response, influencing the spread and severity of disease, according to American research. Around 23.9 days of work were lost on average in 2017 by people affected by stress, according to the Health Executive Agency.

WHY ARE WE SO STRESSED?

People come to TRE from many different situations, whether they've experienced childhood trauma or are simply overwhelmed by a busy

You can shake out to music as well.

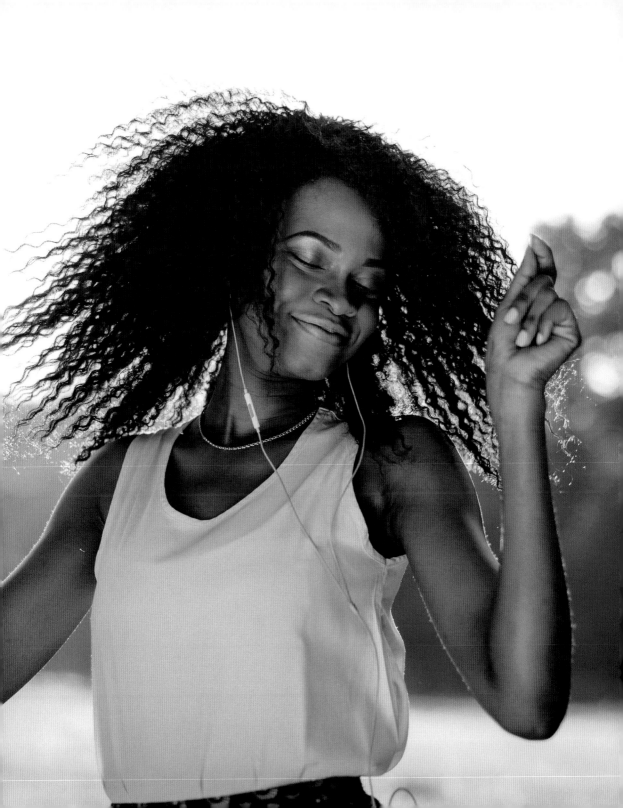

life. There's no doubt that our hyper-connected world has led to more of us missing out on sleep and struggling to confine work to the hours of 9–5. 'Sadly, many people have had adverse experiences in childhood, which have left them primed to react to situations in a certain way. Even if that's not the case for you, the world is a stressful place. A few decades ago there was minimal choice when you went to buy food, but now you've got 15 varieties of rice to choose between,' says Steve. 'Our brains didn't evolve to process that much information. It's easy to feel overwhelmed.'

HOW CAN SHAKING HELP?

When your life feels exhausting or if you've experienced a traumatic event, your body may go into a 'freeze' response. 'It's where we numb ourselves to outside events,' says Steve. 'Shaking is a natural model to reset your body when it's braced against life. Our brains and our muscles get stuck in a certain state, and this is a way of releasing tension. The good news is that, just as we can turn on this state of high alert very quickly, it's also a quick process to turn it back off again. TRE can provide relief from stress, tension and trauma, stimulate your nervous system, optimise control of your muscles and help you feel reconnected with your body.'

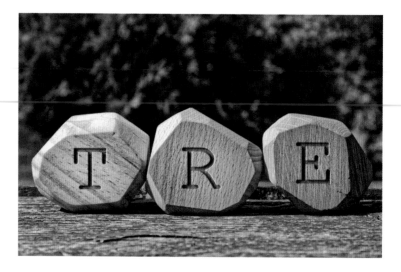

TRE (trauma release exercises) can be a great way to relieve physical stress.

TRY IT AT HOME

'The feeling of shaking is pleasant once you get used to it,' says Steve. 'It should feel effortless and quite curious.' There are seven basic exercises to get the full TRE experience. To get a taster, give these two a try...

STRETCH YOUR LEG

- Stand with your legs spread apart so there is some tension on the inner muscles. Bend forward to touch the ground; you'll feel a stretch on the inner thigh and backs of the legs.

- Slowly walk your hands over to one foot and hold this position for three slow breaths, then walk your hands over to the other foot for three breaths. Walk your hands back to the middle and reach behind through your legs for three breaths. If you feel your legs shaking, just allow it to happen.

OPEN UP YOUR HIPS

- Lie flat on your back, putting the soles of your feet together and let your knees fall open as wide as is comfortable, and relax for a minute.

- Raise your pelvis off the ground about three inches, keeping your knees open. Hold this position for one minute.

- Return to the first position for a minute, close your knees about an inch, and hold for two minutes. Allow any quivering to happen.

- Over time, close your knees another inch and hold for a minute, and then once more. You may find quivering turns into shaking – just allow it to happen.

- Let your feet slide down so you're lying flat. stay there for three minutes and get up slowly.

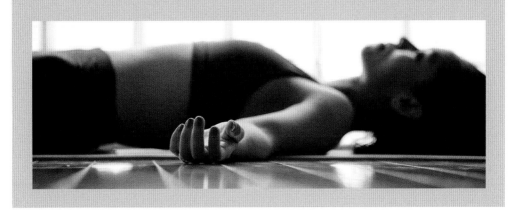

MENOPAUSE FITNESS

You body changes during the menopause so it's good to adjust your workouts. Here's how to target your moves to feel fitter and stronger

If you find it hard to motivate yourself alone, make a date with friends and turn exercise into a social occasion.

THERE'S NO BETTER time to get active and enjoy fitness than when you're going through the menopause. And there's no good reason why you can't throw yourself into the sports and activities you love. The fact your body changes throughout this time simply means you may have to make some minor tweaks to your routine but it needn't spell the end for donning your trainers and working up a sweat – in fact, exercise can even ease many symptoms. 'The menopause affects everyone differently and it's all about working out what's best for you,' says personal trainer Stef Larden. 'One frequent talking point for many women is a fluctuation in energy levels. The best way to deal with it is to make small changes. So if you're running low on energy one day, instead of forcing yourself to go for your usual run, switch to power walking. Or if you usually enjoy a game of tennis, try a doubles match. And if lifting weights is your usual thing, then try bodyweight exercises instead. You'll reap the same rewards and hit the same post-workout high but without exhausting yourself.'

Working out is also an antidote to many menopausal symptoms, including metabolic issues, which can become more prevalent during menopause. A slowing of the metabolism (the rate at which you burn calories) can happen at this time because as you age, you tend to lose muscle mass. Muscles are great calorie burners so as they diminish your metabolism slows down. It makes exercise vital for keeping you trim and healthy. 'I recommend 90–150 minutes of moderate exercise each week,' says Stef. 'This could be as simple as two long walks. Just make sure you go hard enough to work up a sweat and get out of breath.'

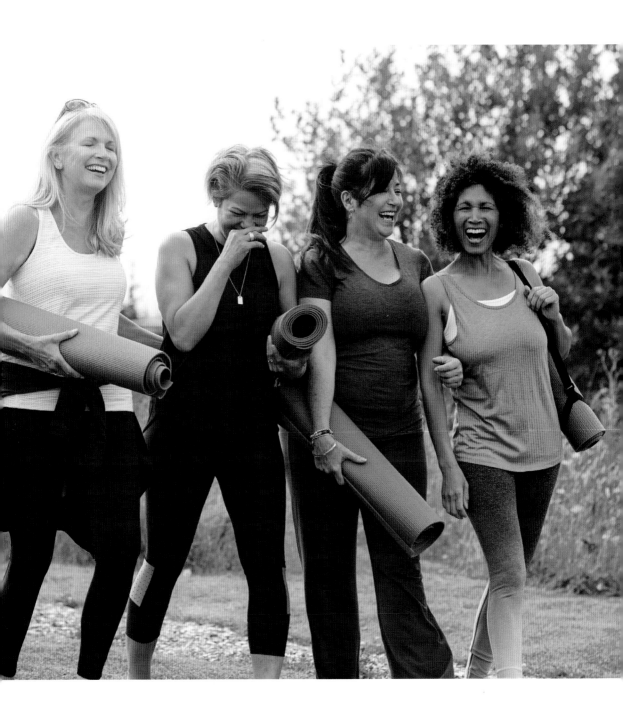

TIGHTENING UP

Menopause exercises must include some work on your pelvic floor. 'Connective tissue can weaken during the menopause (because of the change in hormones) and so does your pelvic floor,' explains Stef. 'These exercises should be non-negotiable in all women's fitness programmes, but particularly when going through the menopause.' There are two kinds of pelvic floor exercise: the first consists of squeezing and releasing the muscles 10–15 times in a row. The second is to squeeze and hold the muscles for a few seconds, as if trying to stop urinating. Then inhale and exhale slowly while keeping them held. 'Spend a few minutes doing each of these two or three times a day to keep your floor strong,' says Stef.

STAYING SUPPLE

Simple stretches during the day can be just as valuable as a hard-core workout. 'Maintaining mobility in your joints and stretching your muscles helps you stay supple and strong, particularly if you have to endure long days of sitting still, commuting or working at a computer as this can leave you feeling stiff and achy,' says Stef. 'Take time each day for stretching exercises, such as rolling your shoulders, circling your wrists and relaxing your body down through each vertebra until your fingertips touch the floor.' Balance is another thing we must hold on to as we get older and practise it regularly. 'Doing squats and lunges will help with balance and core stability – I recommend ten of each three times a day.'

MAINTAINING STRENGTH

'Strength training using weights or resistance is a wonderful way to protect your bones and keep them strong,' says Stef. 'Decreasing oestrogen levels can mean a decrease in bone density, which can lead to osteoporosis. However, workouts using weights, such as 3–4kg dumbbells, or bodyweight exercises – such as squats and the plank – stimulate bone growth. Impact exercises such as running and jumping also help to strengthen your bones, but if you have symptoms of osteoporosis you may be advised against high-octane activities. This doesn't mean you need to avoid all cardio though. Instead, try building it into everyday life. Getting off a stop early on the bus or using the stairs rather than the lift all counts.

FLAT-BELLY MOVES

Feeling more 'apple-shaped' is common during menopause. Your distribution of fat tends to change as you age and the decreased oestrogen levels may play a role in this. But these three moves will help to burn fat, strengthen your core and tone your stomach. Each one should be done for 40 seconds with a 20-second rest and repeated five times.

SQUAT TO CALF RAISE

- Stand with your feet hip-width apart.
- Squat down into a deep squat, then power up so you're on the balls of your feet, lifting your arms into the air as you do so.
- Then, come back down into a squat and repeat.
- Add 3–4kg dumbbells to the move if you can, as this will work your arms at the same time and challenge you.

LUNGE AND SHOULDER PRESS

- Stand with your feet together holding a weight just above your shoulders, out to the side, with elbows bent and your palms facing towards you.
- Step one foot forward and lower your body until your knees are bent 90 degrees, pressing the weight above your head as you do so.
- Move the weight to the other hand and return to the start position as you push back to standing and repeat on the other leg.

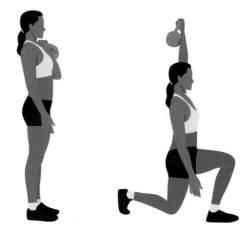

MOUNTAIN CLIMBERS

- Start off in a traditional plank position with your core engaged.
- Bring your right knee forward under your chest, with your toes just off the ground.
- Return to your basic plank. Switch legs, bringing your left knee forward.
- Keep switching your legs and pick up the pace until it feels a little like running in a plank position.

Aim for a moderate exercise level – when you feel out of breath but are able to speak in short sentences. If you can only give one-word answers, you're working too hard. If you can have a full-blown conversation, you're not working hard enough!

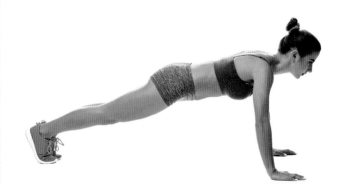

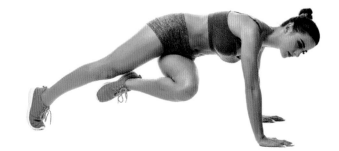

BEATING DIABETES

Find out how to keep your blood sugar in check with food, fitness, supplements and lifestyle.

TO SHAKE OR NOT TO SHAKE?

They're popular and simple to use, but protein shakes cause a spike in insulin because they are absorbed into your blood far more quickly than food protein such as chicken or eggs. So, don't rely on them to sustain you throughout the day – go for protein-based meals instead.

Top tip

Lessen the effect of any carbohydrates in your meal by eating most of the protein first, as this will help to slow the absorption of the carbs.

A NATURAL ALTERNATIVE

To tackle your blood sugar, look to the plant compound berberine – several studies have shown it is as effective at lowering blood glucose as the drug metformin, but without the negative side effects.

MAKE TIME TO CHILL

When under stress, your body's need for glucose increases, so it pumps out cortisol to trigger the release of glycogen: your body's stored sugar. However, too much glycogen is damaging if it's not used up by your muscles, which it won't be if you're just sitting still at a computer or worrying while watching TV. This is why dedicated relaxation time is so important for balanced blood sugar.

DID YOU KNOW...
Adding vinegar or lemon juice to your meals helps reduce the effect the food has on your blood sugar? Try drizzling them over salads and carb-rich veggies, or have half a teaspoon of either in a glass of water, 30 minutes before you eat.

30 g is the amount of fibre you should aim to eat each day. Fibre reduces your risk of developing type 2 diabetes, as it slows the rate at which food is converted into sugar

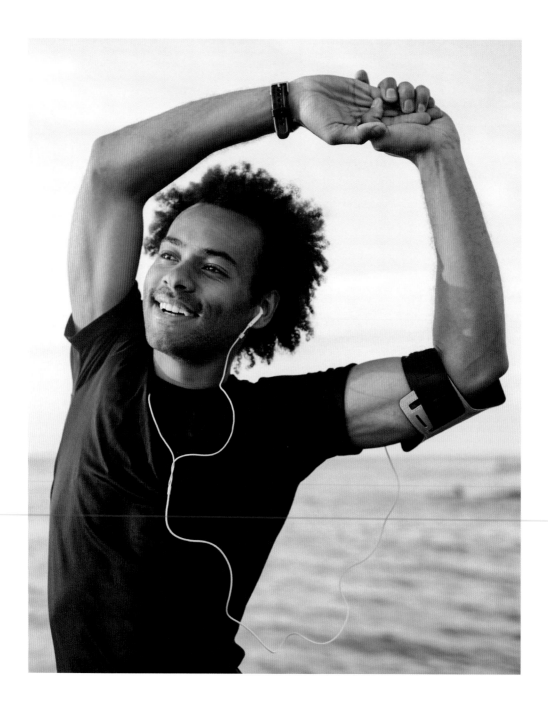

Try it

When you feel yourself starting to tense up and feel anxious, stop what you are doing, put your hands into your lap and let your shoulders drop. Take a long deep breath in through your nose, then when it feels comfortable to do so, i.e. don't force anything, release the breath through pursed lips – this extends the out breath, which is good, as breathing out fully helps relax you.

MIGHTY MINERALS

Chromium can help you manage your blood sugar by increasing insulin sensitivity. It activates an enzyme called tyrosine kinases, which helps insulin to better attach to receptor sites in cells, improving sensitivity to insulin and getting more glucose out of your bloodstream.

TIME TO SLEEP

Lack of sleep leads to higher levels of cortisol and therefore increased glycogen. This is why lack of sleep tends to make you crave sweet things – and it also tells your body to increase the hormone ghrelin, which also tells you to eat more!

Try it

Take a magnesium supplement before bed – look for magnesium threonate (a salt of magnesium combined with L-Threonate), as this has been proven to help reduce anxiety and improve sleep quality.

Add plenty of butter to your baked potatoes … the fat reduces the speed the carbs in the potato are broken down and absorbed

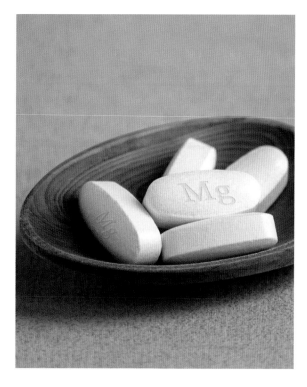

Magnesium can help you sleep more deeply.

FIGHTING FIT

Learn how to train properly to boost your immune system and stay healthy

Running, lifting, twisting; whatever your exercise of choice, no doubt you don your workout gear as often as you can —even when rain sheets down from a gloomy sky — because you hope it's going to keep you healthy. Along with eating well and good quality kip, exercise is a key component of a healthy body and strong immune system. Or is it? It turns out the link between your immune system and the exercise you do could be something of a double-edged sword. While a sedentary lifestyle may hinder health, training too hard can have the same effect.

'Exercise works on multiple levels to keep your immunity strong,' says immunologist Dr Jenna Macciochi (drjennamacciochi.com). 'It

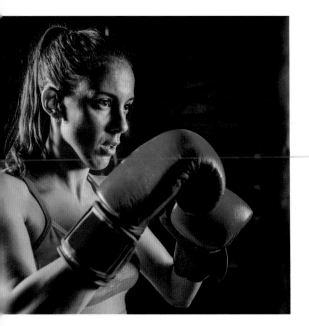

starts by giving your lymphatic system a good old boost and moving lymph fluid – packed with immune cells – around your body. Unlike blood vessels, your lymphatics don't have the luxury of the heart to help them flow and instead rely on muscle movements.' Moving your immune cells around your body helps them perform important surveillance jobs as they seek out infections and potentially spot early development of cancerous cells to squash them before they progress.

'Moving your muscles also produces special immune communication molecules called cytokines, which help rejuvenate your immune system, keeping it young. This is especially important, as after your mid-twenties your thymus gland – where certain immune cells are made – starts to shrink, but moderate exercise helps to actually slow this shrinking process,' says Dr Macciochi. This means if you're an active 70-year-old you could, in theory, be younger (in immune terms) than your sedentary 30-something counterparts! 'Finally, regular, moderate exercise also helps to reduce inflammation, which can be damaging to your tissues if it hangs around too long.'

FIND THAT 'SWEET SPOT'

'Getting your workout regime just right can be a challenge,' says Dr Macciochi. 'People who do little-to-no exercise and have a sedentary lifestyle are generally more likely to pick up infections than those who exercise regularly.' However, it can be just as damaging to overdo it. People who hit the gym five to six times a week and then have to juggle a family or a job on top could be damaging their immune systems. While it's true this system needs exercise to thrive, it also needs adequate rest, recuperation and recovery time. Overworking your body causes stress hormones, such as cortisol and adrenalin, to rise, so it's essential to get some much-needed downtime. 'Everyone is different, and it's important to know what's right for you, but as a general rule, regular, moderate exercise will include three or four varied workout sessions per week, consisting of aerobic, anaerobic and resistance exercises,' says Dr Macciochi.

EXERCISING WHEN UNDER THE WEATHER

Many people adopt a 'keep going' attitude when it comes to illness, but sometimes you need to take a step back and spot when your body is trying to tell you something. 'When you're sick, your immune response

IMMUNE-BOOSTING EXERCISES

- **Walking**. This is the perfect workout; it keeps your body moving, while not putting it under too much strain. Upping your pace and adding some hills will really get your lymphatics pumping.

- **Strength training.** Using weights is very important. Good muscle mass helps to keep your immunity strong, plus you naturally lose muscle as you age – particularly if you don't use it. It's not about lifting heavy weights and building huge muscles, but simply retaining and strengthening what you already have.

- **Swimming**. This aerobic exercise also adds that element of resistance training as you push against the water, while taking the pressure off your joints. It's a little easier on your body than a vigorous run around the park and a perfect immune-booster.

actually signals to your brain to change your behaviour and adopt what are known as "sickness behaviours"', says Dr Macciochi.

This is why you don't feel like getting out of bed when you have flu. In today's modern world we're often focused on 'powering through', but it's very important to pay attention to what your body is telling you. Immune responses are costly and draining, so working out when you're ill can mean less energy available to recover. That said, it does depend on what sort of illness you have. As a general rule of thumb, stick to the following guidelines.'

- If you have a mild head cold, exercise should be fine. In fact, some movement, such as a gentle walk, might even help and will allow your body to squeeze out any remaining bugs and dead cells after fighting infection.

- If you have a fever, you should always rest up and recover.

- If you decide you are going to work out, even if you're not on top form, always moderate it a bit. For example, opt for a gentle walk rather than a fast run, or do yoga rather than aerobics, and choose shorter classes so you don't overload your system. It's also important to start slowly when you get back to your workout schedule after being unwell.

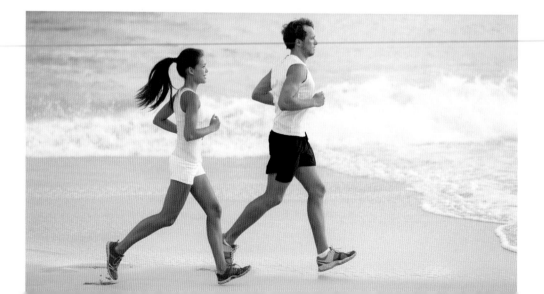

STAND TALL, LOOK YOUNGER

Poor posture can make you look and feel much older and lead to back, neck and shoulder pain, as well as saggy boobs. Here's how to improve your posture

Anyone can develop bad posture. Those who sit at a desk for hours are often thought to be at risk, but you can be standing up and still slouch. If you do have a desk job and tend to slouch over the keyboard, over time you may end up with a rounded upper back, a tight chest and weak upper back muscles. Try not to slump in the chair and make sure your lower back is fully supported. Try not to poke your head forward when looking at your computer screen or slouch from the upper body. If your job involves standing, make sure your shoulders are above your hips and your upper body isn't slouched forwards.

MOBILE HELL

Many of us use mobile devices and excessive use can lead to neck pain. 'Text Neck' is a term coined by chiropractor Dr Dean L Fishman to describe overuse and repetitive strain injury to the neck. Our heads weigh around 10–12 lb (4.5–5.5 kg) and, as you look down at your phone, the weight on your neck increases. Just dropping your neck by a 30-degree angle increases the weight on your neck to 40 lb (18 kg). This can lead to head, neck and even arm pain. So always take regular breaks from texting and looking at your mobile device.

HOW POOR POSTURE AGES YOU...

Why does poor posture make you look and feel older? Here are a few good reasons.

Being aware of your posture and adding support to your chair where needed can help to alleviate back problems.

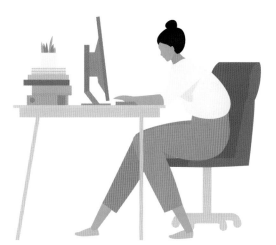

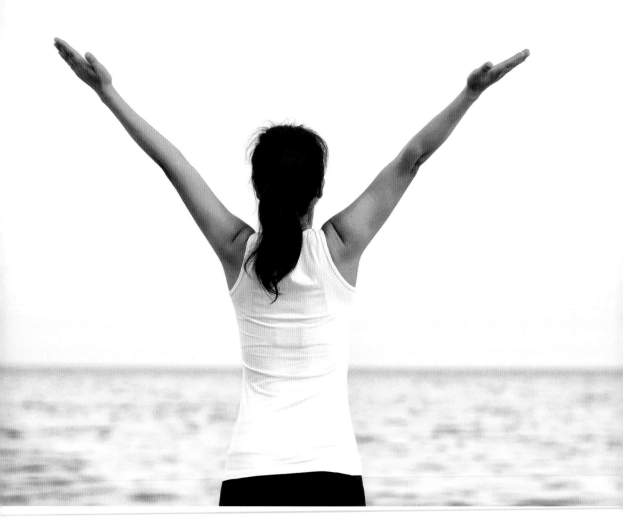

JOINTS AND MUSCLES ARE AFFECTED

You may not realise it, but when your posture is poor, your body is struggling to support you in positions that aren't natural. Muscles may be doing a job they weren't designed for. Over time, slouching and poor posture in general can lead to damage to strained joints and muscles. Bad posture can lead to tight and aching muscles – especially in the back and neck.

RANGE OF MOTION IS REDUCED

If you have poor posture your muscles can be stretched or shortened over time because your body gets used to being permanently slouched.

BACK AND NECK PAIN IS INCREASED

Lower back pain is often caused by poor posture and it can also cause neck pain. When slouching in front of a computer screen, it's easy to poke your head forward, putting a strain on the neck.

BREATHING IS HARDER

Bad posture can also affect your breathing. When you slouch, it constricts the respiratory muscles, including the diaphragm. This means the muscles can't expand properly and you end up taking shallow breaths. This can affect your circulation and also make exercise seem much harder. So when you run, or do any other form of cardio exercise, make sure you stand as tall as possible to give your ribcage a chance to expand properly and allow more air in.

YOU LOOK BIGGER

When you slouch, your shoulders hunch forward and your stomach protrudes. This can make your stomach look bigger than it really is and no amount of dieting or cardio exercise can compensate for poor posture! Simply put, standing tall will make you look thinner.

YOU LOOK OLDER

When you slouch you will look more like an older person – it can add years to your appearance. Also, the more rounded your shoulders, the more your boobs sag. To improve your posture when sitting down, try to keep your head up, your shoulders back and your chest out. Pull your stomach in.

Improving your posture helps you to avoid pain and look slimmer and younger!

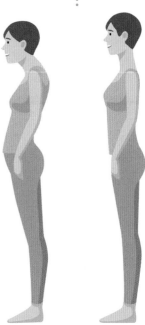

IMPROVE YOUR POSTURE

Try these exercises to improve your posture. Aim to do them twice a week and you'll soon notice your posture begin to change.

- Keep your weight down – the more weight you carry, especially around the middle of your body, the more this will pull on your back and cause weak stomach muscles.

- Exercise regularly – yoga is good, as it will keep your muscles flexible, while resistance training will strengthen your muscles, which will help you maintain good posture.

- Try to stand and sit tall – when sitting at your desk, make sure you are not rounding your shoulders and slouching. When standing, have your shoulders over your hips. When you are standing up, keep your shoulders back and relaxed, pull your stomach in and place your feet about hip-width distance apart, aiming to have your weight evenly on both feet. Imagine a string attached to the top of your head pulling you up.

- Be aware of your posture – it's difficult to have great posture all the time, but it's definitely possible to be aware of your posture. Always correct your posture when you feel like you are starting to slouch.

POSTURE EXERCISES

Improving your posture will help you look younger and slimmer as you'll be able to stand tall and avoid a stooped look.

REACH AND SQUAT
AREAS TRAINED: Thighs, bottom, shoulders, back, core

TECHNIQUE: Stand with your feet slightly wider than shoulder-width apart with your toes turned out to a 45-degree angle. Hold a stability ball with both hands in front of your body. Bend your knees to perform a squat and hold the position. Lift the stability ball with straight arms above your head. Squeeze your shoulder blades and keep your core contracted. Lower the ball and straighten your legs. Perform two sets of ten repetitions.

Be safe
Don't arch your back when lifting the ball overhead.

SEATED LEG RAISES
AREAS TRAINED: Core, side muscles, back

TECHNIQUE: Sit on the stability ball with your arms relaxed next to your sides. Place your feet hip-width apart with your feet directly underneath your knees. Contract your core and lengthen your spine to sit tall. Lift one foot off the floor. Extend your leg. Bend your leg and replace your foot on the floor. Repeat on the other leg. Perform two sets of ten repetitions on each side.

Be safe

If you struggle with balance, hold on to the ball. If you want to make it harder, extend your arms sideways.

BALL BRIDGES

AREAS TRAINED: Core, back, bottom, rear thighs

TECHNIQUE: Lie with your head and shoulders supported on a stability ball. Place your hands on your ribcage and your feet on the floor, hip-width apart. Contract your core muscles to aid your balance. Lower your bottom towards the floor. Lift your hips up until you form a straight line between your shoulders, hips and knees. Perform two sets often to 15 repetitions.

Be safe

Ensure the ball doesn't roll back and forth. Keep it still.

Using a stability ball can help with a variety of exercises to improve your posture and general strength.

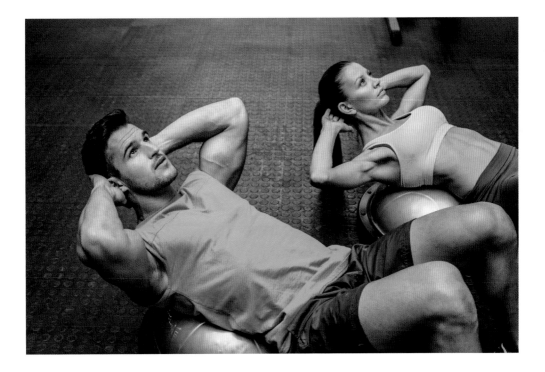

BALL ROLL-OUT
AREAS TRAINED: Core, stomach, side muscles, back, shoulders

TECHNIQUE: Lie with your chest and stomach on a stability ball. Place your elbows and forearms on the ball underneath your chest. Position your shoulders directly over your elbows. Keep your feet hip-width or slightly wider apart. Lift your body off the ball into a plank position. Push your elbows forward to roll the ball away from you. Don't let your hips drop. Pull your elbows back in underneath your shoulders. Ensure that your body doesn't rock forwards and backwards. Perform two sets of ten repetitions.

Be safe

If this is too hard, keep your knees on the floor.

WIDE ROW
AREA TRAINED: Upper back

TECHNIQUE: Lie with your chest and stomach on a stability ball. Hold a weight in each hand on the floor with your palms facing your feet. Lift the weights level with your shoulders. Squeeze your shoulder blades together. Hold the position for a count of two before lowering the weights. Perform two sets of ten repetitions.

Be safe

Keep your body still — only your arms should be doing the movement.

BACK EXTENSION WITH SHOULDER PRESS
AREAS TRAINED: Back, core, neck, shoulders

TECHNIQUE: Lie with your stomach and hips supported on a stability ball. Support your feet against a secure object or wall. Keep your arms at right angles with your hands next to your shoulders, palms facing down. Lift your head, shoulders and arms until parallel to the floor. Extend your arms out in front of you, squeezing your shoulder blades. Bring your arms back and lower your upper body. Perform two sets of ten repetitions.

Be safe

Don't lift your upper body up too high.

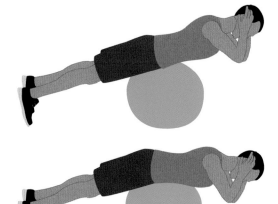

RESISTANCE BAND BALL CRUNCHES

AREAS TRAINED: Core, stomach muscles

TECHNIQUE: Tie a resistance band around a pole or secure object about the height of your stability ball. Lie with the small of your back supported on the stability ball. Hold the edges of the resistance band next to your ears. Crunch your head and shoulders off the ball. Slowly lower with control, ensuring you keep tension on your resistance band. Perform two sets of ten repetitions.

Be safe

Keep your upper back on the ball to make the exercise easier.

PRONE ROTATIONS

AREAS TRAINED: Back, chest, shoulders, side muscles

TECHNIQUE: Lie on your stomach on a stability ball resting your hands and feet on the floor. Lift one arm and rotate it up to the ceiling. Look up towards your hand. Aim to have a straight line between your arms. Hold for a count of two. Lower with control and repeat on the other side. Perform two sets of eight to ten repetitions on each side.

Be safe

Keep your legs slightly wider than hip-width apart to aid your balance.

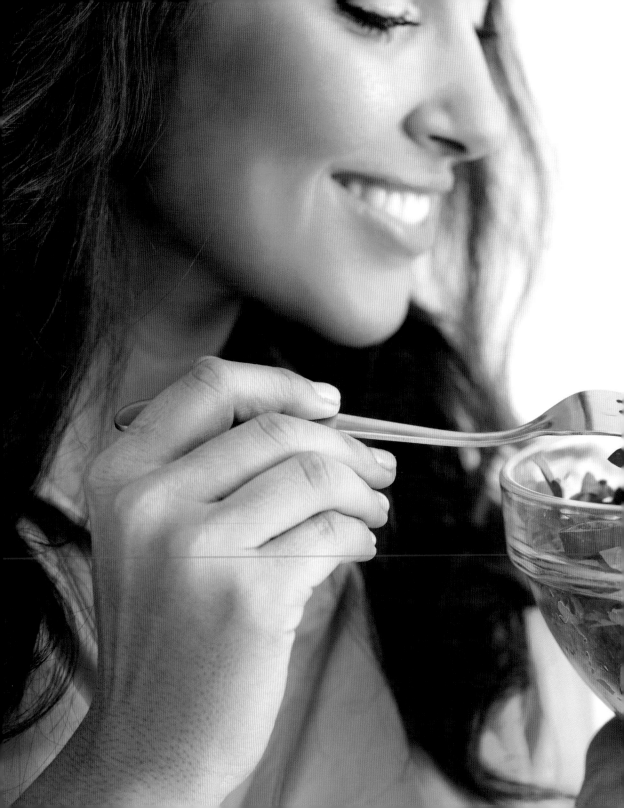

FEED
YOUR BODY

The food you eat is as important to how you function as any other part of your lifestyle. Look at your diet and work out how you can make small tweaks for a big difference in how you feel.

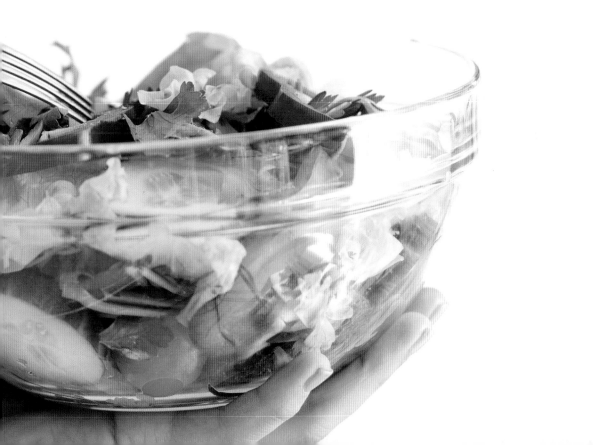

GOLDEN RULES OF FOOD

Follow our simple guidelines to eat better, train harder,
store less fat and lose weight

FOCUS ON GOOD FATS

'Eating fatty foods makes you fat' may sound like a logical assumption,
but it's a bit more complicated than that. It is true that at nine
calories per gram, fat is more calorific than carbohydrate or
protein – which contain four calories per gram – but certain fats
are a crucial part of your diet. The mono- and polyunsaturated fats that
occur naturally in foods, such as oily fish, nuts, seeds, olives and coconut
oil, for example, play key roles in boosting metabolism, improving
hormone synthesis and increasing 'good' HDL cholesterol. Don't be
fooled by 'low-fat' options, either. Most have been highly processed to
remove the fat and tend to be packed with salt and sugar to enhance
their flavour. Instead, focus your energies on avoiding processed junk
foods, high in unhealthy man-made trans fats, and enjoy daily servings of
healthy, naturally occurring fat sources.

VEG OUT

All fruit and veg contain health-enhancing nutrients. But while the
five-a-day mantra is good at encouraging people to eat more
fresh produce in general, if you want to get the most out of your
training and support your fat-burning and muscle-building
efforts, you need to be a lot more specific about your intake of
these important foods. For a start, try to have as much veg as
possible, while cutting back on fruit. Some fruits are very high
in fructose, a type of sugar that plays havoc with blood sugar
levels, making you far more likely to store fat. Vegetables, on the
other hand, contain no fructose, but are just as nutrient dense,
so it makes sense to eat more veggies than fruit. Green vegetables
in particular are a great choice – they're an excellent source of slow-

release carbs, unlike starchy root vegetables, such as potatoes, which can also negatively affect your blood sugar levels. Eat as many servings of green veg as possible each day and limit your fruit intake to one or two servings, ideally from low-sugar sources such as blueberries, raspberries or strawberries.

STAY WHOLESOME

Nothing will hamper your progress more than overindulging in processed foods. Regularly eating refined carbs and sugars that form the basis of most processed snacks, baked goods and fast foods will sap your energy levels and cause fat-storing blood sugar spikes, making it far harder to lose weight or perform at an optimum level. To make matters worse, these foods typically contain high levels of man-made trans fats, which will make you feel even more lethargic and boost your levels of 'bad' LDL cholesterol. For a healthier alternative, swap processed foods for more naturally indulgent wholefood alternatives. For example, trade crisps for nuts, chocolate spread for peanut butter, and sugary breakfast cereal for porridge oats, all of which have additional nutritional benefits.

CURB CALORIE-COUNTING

It's easy to fall into the trap of focusing on the quantity of calories you're eating, especially if you're trying to lose weight. But the quality of the food is far more important, because calories alone don't provide a reliable indication of the effect a food can have on your metabolism. For example, consuming a can of fizzy drink – which will send your blood sugar soaring – is far more damaging to your fat-loss efforts than eating two protein-rich poached eggs, despite the fact that both contain a similar number of calories. It's also easy to use calorie counting as an excuse to justify poor food choices – a 'healthy' packet of crisps may contain fewer than 100 calories, but it's likely to be full of trans fats and other nasties. Instead of getting hung up on how many calories every item of food contains, concentrate on eating plenty of wholefoods, vegetables and high-quality protein.

PICK PROTEIN

Protein plays a crucial role in building muscle, but it's easy to underestimate just how much you need to maximise its benefits. Research into the metabolic demands for protein varies greatly, with studies suggesting anything from 0.8 g per kg of bodyweight to over 2 g as a daily guideline. If you want to keep things simple, aim to eat a 20–25 g serving of protein – good sources of which include meat, fish, beans, pulses and eggs – with every meal, including breakfast. But if you're struggling to achieve that, adding an extra post-workout serving on training days can be a good way to help meet your daily protein goal. In addition to aiding your muscle-building efforts, protein-rich foods also tend to have a high satiety value, making you less likely to have the urge to pig out between meals. That said, try to eat lean protein. Red meat is an excellent source of protein, but certain cuts are very fatty and high in calories. Too much saturated fat can promote inflammation – not great for anyone leading an active lifestyle, especially if you're prone to injuries. Cut back on pies, pastries, biscuits and chocolate, and increase your intake of lean protein.

DON'T CUT OUT ALL CARBS

Drastically cutting carbs is likely to leave you feeling tired and unable to perform at your best. Too much in your diet and your body will dump the excess as fat, making it harder to shift that weight. If you're looking to lose some weight, reduce your intake to one to two portions a day and focus on including these before and after training. For the rest of the day, base your meals around half a plate of vegetables plus a little starchy veg, such as butternut squash, sweet potato and plenty of protein.

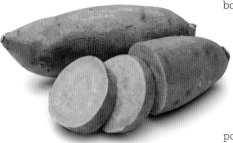

INCLUDE THESE HEALTHY and delicious foods in your diet...

Quinoa

Quinoa contains almost three times the amount of (complete) protein and it's a complex carbohydrate to boot. This means it's perfect for padding out lunchtime salads and keeping tummy rumbles at bay well into the afternoon. Buy it ready cooked for speed and convenience.

Avocado

Poor old fat has been demonised for far too long. Not only do we need fat to burn fat, but it also keeps your brain happy and is the king of

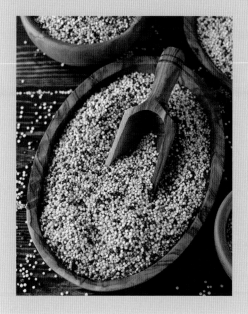

satiety. One study published in *Nutrition Journal* proved that those who had half an avocado with lunch were 40 per cent less hungry for two hours afterwards.

Lentils

Chewing a tablespoon of lentils takes some time – so imagine how long they take to digest! This is due to their high fibre content and, put simply, they will keep you fuller for longer. Lentils are a high-density, low-calorie food – making them weight-loss friendly. Not to mention that they are also loaded with energy-producing iron – essential for those extra gym sessions!

Brown rice

An easy way to lower the GI of your meal and level out your blood sugar is to simply swap out fluffy, white rice for its nuttier counterpart. Brown rice is what your white rice used to look like before it was stripped of its fibrous hull. It's far fleshier than white rice when it comes to nutritional value, too, as it's rich in B vitamins and minerals such as calcium, magnesium and potassium.

Eggs

Eggs are nutrient powerhouses and one of the best sources of protein around, sitting up high on the Satiety Index scale. Hard-boiled eggs are the perfect, pre-packaged snack.

MAXIMISE YOUR CALORIE BURN

Want to burn more calories? It's easier than you think ...

UP YOUR PROTEIN

Stay fuller for longer by making it a habit to build your meal around protein. When the stomach breaks up protein, the peptides that are released send a message to the brain telling it you are full. Genius! Add beans and pulses to salads and casseroles or lean meat to lunches and dinners.

Adding protein such as grilled chicken to a salad greatly boosts its energy value.

BAN THE BOOZE

Hold back on a glass of wine at dinner and you'll save 150 calories; cut back on more and you'll feel far less bloated. It will also save you a lot of sugar and empty calories and give your liver a rest so it can metabolise calories and burn fat instead.

EAT MORE FAT

Yes, you heard us right! But not all fats are equal. Choose natural fats found in nuts, seeds, oils, fish and avocados and they will stop you from feeling hungry and you won't snack or overeat. Good fat also burns fat by shifting it out of fat cells and into the bloodstream where

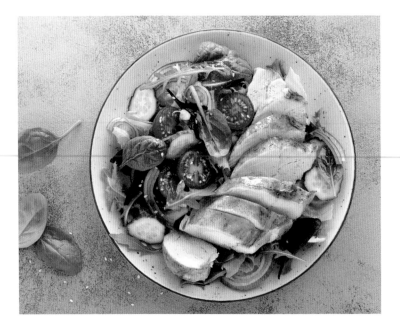

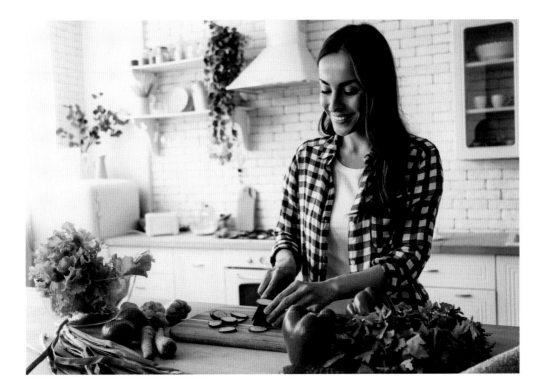

it can be burned off. Try drizzling olive, hemp, sesame, nut or avocado oil onto salads.

DROP THE JUNK

Aim to prepare and cook as many of your own meals from scratch as possible. This way you'll avoid eating unhealthy processed foods, unnecessary calories, artificial ingredients, preservatives and hidden fats and salts.

ADD SOME EXTRA GOODNESS

Get more dietary fibre into your day by sprinkling psyllium seed husks on your breakfast or in smoothies. Their fibre content can reduce appetite and improve digestion.

Prepare from scratch to avoid eating too much processed food.

YOUR FIT FOR LIFE MEAL PLAN

Incorporate these healthy recipes into your diet and you'll
stay fitter, healthier and stronger for longer

This food plan includes 28 healthy recipe ideas for each mealtime:
breakfast, lunch and dinner. This means you can mix and match your
favourites for the next four weeks — and longer if you want to! From
homemade cereal and breakfast smoothies to Moroccan couscous
salads and tortillas with salmon, there's something to tickle all taste
buds. Incorporating our healthy food plan into your life couldn't be
easier; not only are the recipes easy to follow and delicious, but you
can cook for family and friends, too, so there will be no effort involved
in trying to make different meals for everyone! The combination of
meals will help you reduce your calorie intake by the recommended
amount for safe weight-loss. So, all you need to do now is choose what
you want to eat for your first week and take our list with you when you
do your weekly shop and get cooking! It's a tasty and nutritious plan
designed to help you get the bikini body you've always wanted. Who
said that losing weight means you have to give up the foods that you
love? Enjoy!

BREAKFAST RECIPES

Porridge and yoghurt

145 g/5 oz bowl of porridge oats made with 125ml/¼ pint of semi-
skimmed milk, cooked to pack instructions and served with 1tbsp
of natural bio yoghurt in the middle.
Per serving: cals 116 | fat 5.1 g | sat fat 2 g | protein 4.8 g

Egg and soldiers

1 boiled egg with 1 slice of wholemeal toast and light olive spread.
Per serving: cals 200 | fat 11 g | sat fat 3.6 g | protein 14.8 g

Breakfast in a pan (serves 4 – weekend treat!)

Heat a medium non-stick frying pan, add 4 pork chipolata sausages and fry for 3 mins. Add 4 rashers bacon, turning occasionally, and cook for about 5 mins. Add 140g button mushrooms and cook for a further 3–5 mins. Drain any excess fat and arrange the ingredients so they are evenly spread out. Beat 6 eggs and season, then add to the pan, swirling to fill the spaces. Gently move with a fork for 2 mins over a low-medium heat until beginning to set. Scatter over 8 halved cherry tomatoes, then grill for 2 mins until set. Cut into wedges and serve.

Per serving: cals 349 | fat 26 g | sat fat 8 g | protein 25 g

Berry smoothie

Slice 1 small, ripe banana into a blender or food processor and add 140 g /5 oz blackberries, blueberries, raspberries or strawberries (or use a mix of all four). Whizz until smooth and then, while the blades are still whirring, pour in as much apple juice or mineral water to dilute the mix and make the consistency you like.

Per serving: cals 123 | fat 0 g | sat fat 0 g | protein 2 g

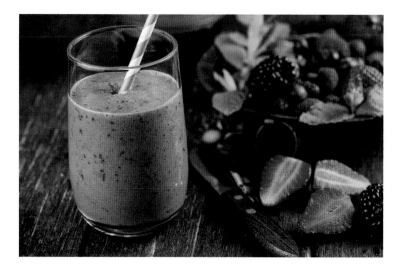

You can make delicious berry smoothies using whatever berries are currently in season.

Muesli with blueberries

Pour 30 g/1 oz of unsweetened muesli into a bowl and top with 1 tbsp of blueberries and 125 ml/¼ pint of semi-skimmed milk.

Per serving: cals 161 | fat 8.1 g | sat fat 1.6 g | protein 4.8 g

Melon, kiwi, grape and papaya salad (serves 2)

Cut 1 ripe cantaloupe melon in half across the middle and deseed, then scoop out the melon flesh into melon balls or chunks and add to a large bowl for mixing. Chop up 3 peeled kiwis, a handful of green grapes and 1 large peeled and deseeded papaya (you can leave the grapes whole if you'd prefer) and add them to the bowl. Stir and spoon into the melon halves — saves on the washing up! Experiment with different melons and seasonal fruits such as strawberries.

Per serving: cals 101 | fat 0.6 g | sat fat 0 g | protein 2 g

You could add a few strawberries to enliven this salad.

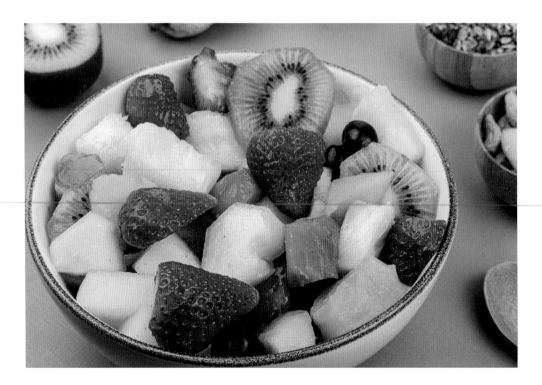

Homemade cereal

Mix 300 g/10.5 oz jumbo oats, 100 g/3.5 oz bran cereal, 25g/1 oz wheatgerm, 100 g/3.5 oz walnut pieces, 100 g/3.5 oz raisins, 140 g/5 oz dried apricots, snipped into chunks and 50 g/2 oz sunflower seeds in a large cereal container. Serve 30 g/1 oz with 125 ml/0.2 pint semi-skimmed milk.
Per serving: cals 124 | fat 3 g | sat fat 0 g |protein 4 g

Scrambled eggs and ham

Scramble 2 medium-sized eggs with a dash of skimmed milk and add seasoning to taste. Serve with 2 slices of good-quality lean ham.
Per serving: cals 262 | fat 16.3 g | sat fat 3.5 g | protein 25 g

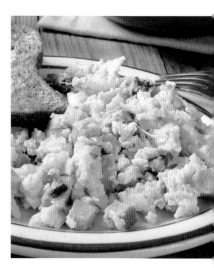

Bran flakes with fruit

140 g/5 oz bowl of bran flakes with 1 chopped apple and 1 sliced banana with 125 ml/¼ pint of semi-skimmed milk.
Per serving: cals 265 | fat 3.5 g | sat fat 1.5 g | protein 8.5 g

Fruit and yoghurt with seeds

Cut up three of your favourite fruits (such as an apple, a pear and a mango) and mix with 3 tbsps of natural bio yoghurt. Sprinkle with 15 g/½ oz toasted pumpkin seeds.
Per serving: cals 225 | fat 1 g | sat fat 0.5 g | protein 10 g

A little grilled ham adds taste and extra protein to scrambled eggs.

Muesli with grated apple

Pour 50 g/2 oz of unsweetened muesli into a bowl and top with 1 apple (peeled and grated) and 125 ml/¼ pint of semi-skimmed milk.
Per serving: cals 350 | fat 5 g | sat fat 1.5 g | protein 10 g

Scrambled eggs with smoked salmon

Scramble 2 medium-sized eggs with 1tsp of low-fat butter and serve with 25 g/1 oz smoked salmon, cut into thin strips.
Per serving: cals 234 | fat 8.6 g | sat fat 1.7 g | protein 8.9 g

Cooked tomatoes on toast

Slice 1 large or 2 small tomatoes thickly and pan-fry in a little olive oil until softened. Sit on top of 1 slice of wholemeal toast with light olive spread and serve.

Per serving: cals 198 | fat 2.5 g | sat fat 0.8 g | protein 9.8 g

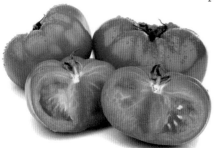

Shredded Wheat

A tasty, healthy cereal without any extra calorie additions from nuts, honey or sugar coating! Simply pour 45 g/1½ oz in a bowl with 125 ml/¼ pint semi-skimmed milk.

Per serving: cals 218 | fat 3.2 g | sat fat 0.3 g | protein 9.6 g

Scrambled eggs on toast

Scramble 2 medium-sized eggs with a dash of skimmed milk and add seasoning to taste. Spoon onto 1 slice of wholemeal toast with light olive spread and serve.

Per serving: cals 324 | fat 3.8 g | sat fat 1.6 g | protein 18.8 g

Muffin and eggs

1 toasted wholemeal muffin, split in 2 and topped with 2 scrambled eggs.

Per serving: cals 318 | fat 3.9 g | Sat fat 1.7 g | Protein 16.5 g

Breakfast fruit smoothie

In a blender, make a smoothie from 250 ml/½ pint semi-skimmed milk, 60 g natural bio yoghurt, 125 g/4½ oz strawberries, 2 passion fruit and 2 tsps honey. Process until the consistency is smooth.

Per serving: cals 205 | fat 4.8 g | sat fat 3 g | protein 6.5 g

Mushrooms on toast

Heat 1 tbsp olive oil in a pan and quickly fry around 50–60 g/1¾–2½ oz thickly sliced mushrooms. Spoon onto 1 slice of wholemeal toast with light olive spread and serve.

Per serving: cals 255 | fat 16.3 g | sat fat 2.8 g | protein 5.6 g

Cooked breakfast

For a special weekend treat, grill 1 lean sausage, 1 rasher bacon,
1 large flat mushroom and 1 tomato cut in half. Serve with 1 poached
egg and 1 slice of wholemeal toast spread with a light olive spread.
Per serving: cals 517 | fat 25 g | sat fat 12.3 g | protein 21.7 g

Wholemeal muffin

Toast 1 wholemeal muffin, cut in half and spread with a light olive
spread
Per serving: cals 145 | fat 3.5 g | sat fat 1 g | protein 8 g

Toast and Marmite

1 slice of wholemeal toast with a light olive spread and Marmite.
Per serving: cals 118 | fat 2.3 g | sat fat 1.3 g | protein 4.6 g

Porridge with yoghurt and honey

Make a bowl of porridge in the microwave or on the
hob with 40 g/1½ oz oats and semi-skimmed milk,
according to pack instructions. Serve with 1 tbsp
natural bio yoghurt in the middle and a little honey.
Per serving: cals 284 | fat 6 g | sat fat 2 g | protein 7.7 g

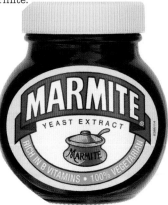

Wholemeal bagel with scrambled eggs

Scramble 2 eggs with 1tsp of low-fat butter and serve on a
warmed wholemeal bagel split in 2.
Per serving: cals 298 | fat 9.6 g | sat fat 2 g | protein 12.3 g

Weetabix

A healthy cereal without any calorie additions from nuts, honey
or sugar coating! Simply serve 2 Weetabix biscuits in a bowl with
125 ml/0.2 pint of semi-skimmed milk.
Per serving: cals 195 | fat 3 g | sat fat 1.5 g | protein 9 g

Bran with fruit and nuts

Mix 40 g/1½ oz of bran flakes or Kellogg's All-Bran with 2–3 chopped dried apricots and 1tsp of chopped toasted walnuts. Serve with 125 ml/¼ pint of semi-skimmed milk.

Per serving: cals 289 | fat 4 g | sat fat 2 g | protein 10 g

Breakfast fruit and veg smoothie

In a blender, make a smoothie from 1 apple, 4 carrots, 2 sticks celery and 2 kiwi fruit. Process until the consistency is smooth and drink straight away.

Per serving: cals 145 | fat 0 g | sat fat 0 g | protein 4 g

Change up the fruits for this salad depending on your mood and what is in season.

Natural yoghurt, fruit and toasted sunflower seeds

Cut up 3 of your favourite fruits (such as a pear, a couple of plums and a few strawberries) and mix with 3 tbsps of low-fat natural bio yoghurt. Sprinkle with 15 g/½ oz toasted sunflower seeds and serve.

Per serving: cals 226 | fat 1 g | sat fat 0.5 g | protein 12 g

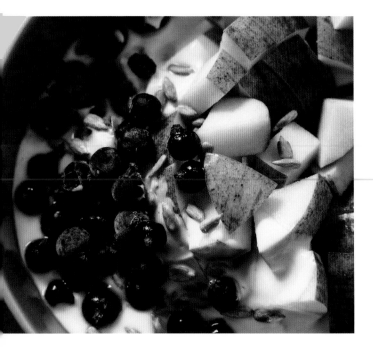

Fruit smoothie

Cut 1 medium mango down either side of the flat stone, then peel and cut the flesh into chunks. Peel and chop 1 banana. Put the mango and banana into a food processor or blender, along with 500ml orange juice. Process until smooth and thick. Keep in the fridge and use the day you make it.

Per serving: cals 107 | fat 1 g | sat fat 0 g | protein 1 g

LUNCH RECIPES

Chicken salad tortilla wrap

Warm 1 wholemeal tortilla wrap and fill
with 3–4 slices of cooked chicken, 1 handful
of shredded lettuce, 1 chopped tomato, a
few slices of cucumber and 1tbsp of low-fat
mayonnaise.
Per serving: cals 242 | fat 3.1 g | sat fat 1.7 g
| protein 18 g

Speedy asparagus tortilla (serves 4)

400 g/14 oz fresh asparagus tips, trimmed
• 10 large eggs, preferably organic • 2 tbsps
butter, melted • 50 g/1¾ oz Manchego
cheese, grated • Salt and black pepper

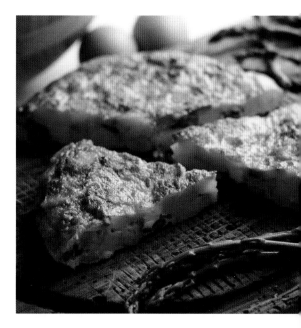

Method

Blanch the asparagus in boiling water for 1 min, then drain and
refresh under cold water. Beat the eggs until light and fluffy and
season with the salt and freshly ground black pepper. Brush 4
individual gratin microwave-proof dishes with the butter. Pour a
quarter of the egg mixture into each dish. Microwave each dish
separately on full power for 1–2 mins until the egg is just set. Preheat
the grill until very hot. Arrange the asparagus over the egg and
scatter over the cheese. Grill for 1 min until golden. Serve with a crisp,
green salad.
Per serving: cals 280 | fat 21 g | sat fat 9 g | protein 34 g

*Asparagus in
season adds a
touch of luxury to
a tortilla.*

Watercress, nectarine and Parma ham salad (serves 4)

For the salad

• 4 ripe but firm nectarines, rinsed • 12 slices Parma ham• 1 x
150 g/5 oz bag salad • 25 g/1 oz chunk Parmesan plus 1 tbsp grated •
Salt and black pepper (optional)

For the dressing
• 4 tbsps single cream • 1 garlic clove, peeled and finely grated • 3 tsps lemon juice

Method
Cut the nectarines into thin slices, removing the stones, and arrange on 4 plates. Place the Parma ham in waves on top of the nectarines then add a handful of salad leaves. Shave the Parmesan over the plates using a potato peeler. To make the dressing, put the grated Parmesan, cream, garlic and lemon juice in a screw top jar and shake well. Taste, then season, if you like. Drizzle over the salad and serve.
Per serving: cals 233 | fat 11 g | sat fat 4.3 g | protein 17 g

Tuna and egg salad
Prepare a mixed salad with chopped lettuce, 6 halved cherry tomatoes, a few slices of cucumber and 6 olives. Place on a plate and drizzle with olive oil. Decorate salad with 1 hard-boiled egg, quartered, and top with a small tin of flaked tuna (in water, not oil).
Per serving: cals 245 | fat 8.5 g | sat fat 2.3 g | protein 39.5 g

Low-fat cream cheese, Ryvita crackers, celery and grapes
Prepare 2 Ryvitas with a liberal spread of cream cheese. Serve with 4–5 sticks of celery and a small bunch of grapes.
Per serving: cals 135 | fat 3.5 g | sat fat 1 g | protein 9 g

You can use other fruits as well as grapes with your cream cheese.

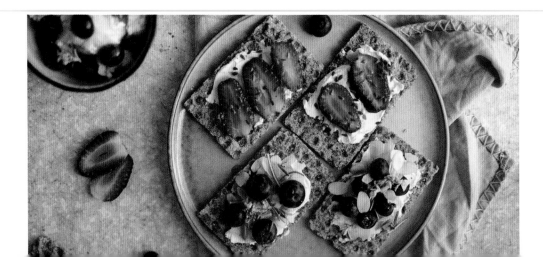

Grilled gammon, poached egg and tomato

Grill 150 g/5 oz lean gammon (cut off any excess fat) and serve with 1 poached egg and 1 grilled tomato.

Per serving: cals 289 | fat 20.3 g | sat fat 4.2 g | protein 31.5 g

Warmed pitta bread filled with cheese salad

Fill 1 warmed pitta bread with a handful of grated Cheddar cheese, 1 thinly sliced tomato, some shredded lettuce and 1 tbsp of low-fat mayonnaise.

Per serving: cals 273 | fat 8.1 g | sat fat 1.2 g | protein 19 g

Moroccan couscous salad with seared lamb (serves 4)

• 175 g/6 oz couscous • 2 oranges • 3 tbsp olive oil • 1tbsp clear honey • 1 tbsp chopped fresh mint • 50 g/1¾ oz raisins or sultanas • 75 g/2½ oz apricots, chopped • 75 g/2½ oz seedless grapes, halved • 1 wedge honeydew melon,cut into small chunks • 25 g/1 oz whole almonds • Handful of mixed salad leaves • 4 x 110 g/4 oz lamb rump or leg steaks • Mint sprigs, to garnish

Just touch the lamb with heat to seal in the flavour.

Method

Put the couscous into a large bowl with a pinch of salt. Pour over enough boiling water to cover, then leave to soak for about 15 mins, until swollen and tender. Peel and segment the oranges, removing all the pith if possible. Put the segments into a bowl, then stir in the honey, olive oil and chopped mint. Fluff up the couscous with a fork, then add the orange mixture, stirring gently. Add the raisins or sultanas, apricots, grapes, melon, almonds and salad leaves, tossing to mix. Share between 4 serving plates or bowls. Heat a chargrill pan or non-stick frying pan. Brush the lamb steaks with 2tbsps olive oil, then chargrill or fry them for 3–4 mins on each side. Wrap them in foil and leave to rest for 4–5 mins, then slice and arrange on top of the salads. Garnish with the sprigs of mint, then serve.

Per serving: cals 285 | fat 7 g | sat fat 1 g | protein 32 g

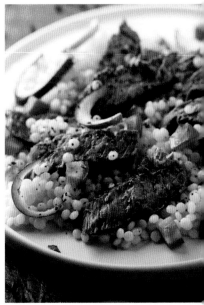

Crab and mango naan club sandwich (serves 4)

• 2 x 170 g/6 oz tins crab meat, well drained • 1 small red chilli, deseeded and finely chopped • 4 tbsps fresh mayonnaise• 2 tbsps lime juice • 2 tbsps finely chopped chives • small garlic and coriander naan breads • 3–4 tbsps mango chutney • 2 large handfuls of wild rocket

Method

Place the crab meat in a bowl with the chilli, mayonnaise and lime juice. Mix well, then stir in the chives. Prepare the naan according to the instructions on the packet and leave to cool. Spread mango chutney two naan breads Arrange the rocket over them and spread crab mixture on top. Place remaining naan breads to form 2 sandwiches. Slice in half and stick a cocktail stick in each half to hold.

Per serving: cals 320 | fat 12 g | sat fat 2 g | protein 19 g

Hot chicken and salad tortilla wrap

Warm 1 wholemeal tortilla wrap and fill with 3–4 slices hot chicken, 1 handful of shredded lettuce, 1 chopped tomato and 1 tbsp of low-fat mayonnaise.

Per serving: cals 242 | fat 3.1 g | sat fat 1.7 g | protein 18 g

Quick to prepare, a wrap makes a perfect easy lunch.

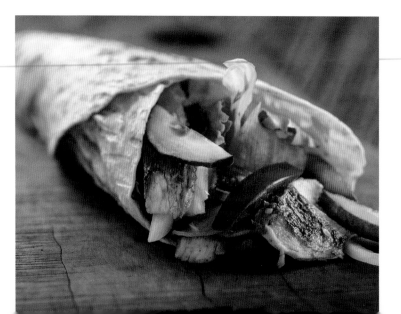

Creamy smoked mackerel sandwich

Skin and flake 125 g/4½ oz smoked mackerel fillets, then mix with 1tsp mayonnaise and 1tsp low-fat natural bio yoghurt. You could add chopped spring onion Spread onto 2 thin slices wholemeal bread and top with crisp lettuce leaves.
Per serving: cals 246 | fat 4.9 g | sat fat 1.8 g | protein 24 g

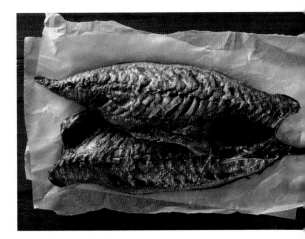

Bagel with scrambled egg

Split a bagel in half and top with 1 scrambled egg.
Per serving: cals 283 | fat 8.5 g | sat fat 3.9 g | protein 14 g

Smoked trout and cucumber open sandwich (serves 2)

Flake 125 g/4½ oz pack skinless, smoked trout fillets into a large bowl, then stir in 125 g/4½ oz quark (or other low-fat soft cheese) and ½ tsp of horseradish sauce to taste. Season with black pepper and lemon juice. Toast 2 slices of granary bread then top each piece with cucumber slices and 25 g/1 oz of watercress. Spoon half the trout pâté on top of each and serve with halved cherry tomatoes on the side.
Per serving: cals 223 | fat 9.2 g | sat fat 2 g | protein 28 g

Ham and salad roll

Choose a normal-size wholemeal roll (rather than a huge bap) and fill with lean ham and salad of your choice. Spread the cut surface of the roll with a small amount of low-fat mayonnaise.
Per serving: cals 275 | fat 5 g | sat fat 1.5 g | protein 13.3 g

Cottage cheese with chives, Ryvita crackers, celery and apple

Top 2 Ryvitas with some cottage cheese with chives. Serve with 2 celery sticks and 1 sliced apple.
Per serving: cals 110 | fat 1.8 g | sat fat 0.9 g | protein 9 g

Filling and versatile, a baked potato can take a great variety of healthy toppings.

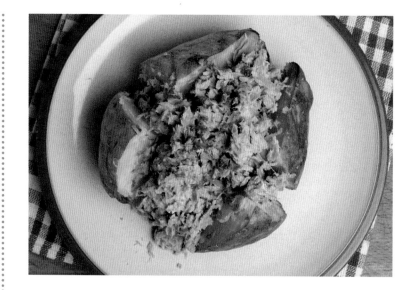

Jacket potato with tuna mayo

Bake or microwave a jacket potato (140 g/5 oz) and top with a 120 g/ 4¼ oz tin of tuna (in water) mixed with 2 tbsps low-fat mayonnaise.
Per serving: cals 298 |fat 1.8 g | sat fat 0.9 g | protein 9.5 g

Cheese and mushroom omelette and green salad

Pan-fry 6 mushrooms (sliced) in an omelette pan with 1tsp of light olive margarine. Then add 2 beaten eggs and make an omelette, sprinkling over 1tbsp grated cheese while cooking. Serve with a small green salad.
Per serving: cals 296 | fat 25 g | sat fat 10.2 g | protein 28 g

Egg and bacon salad

Make a mixed salad with chopped lettuce, 6 halved cherry tomatoes and a few slices of cucumber. Then roughly chop 1 hard-boiled egg and 2 rashers of cooked, crispy bacon, place on top of salad and serve straight away.
Per serving: cals 265 | fat 13 g | sat fat 6 g | protein 32 g

Greek salad (serves 4)

• 4 large ripe tomatoes, each one cut into 8 wedges • ½ a cucumber, chopped into small chunks • ½ an iceberg lettuce, chopped • 20 green or black olives • 350 g/12 oz feta cheese, cubed, 1 red onion if desired. For the dressing • 4 tbsps olive oil • 2tbsps lemon juice

Method

Mix together the tomatoes, cucumber, lettuce, olives and feta cheese. Next, whisk together the olive oil and lemon juice to make the dressing. Toss together and serve with plenty of chopped flat-leaf parsley on top.

Per serving: cals 333 | fat 29 g | sat fat 14 g | protein 18 g

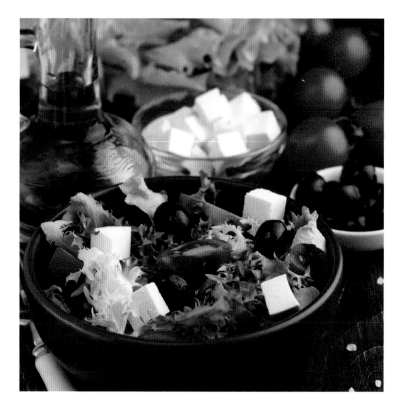

Evoke sun-filled holidays with a refreshing Greek salad.

DINNER RECIPES

Teriyaki salmon (serves 2)
 • 2 x 175 g/6 oz salmon fillets • 8 tbsps teriyaki sauce • 1 small pak choi, washed • 2 carrots, peeled • 50 g/1¾ oz baby corn • 1 celery stick • 1 tsp sesame oil • ½ lemon

Method
Put the salmon fillets into a plastic food bag, then pour in the teriyaki sauce and shake gently. Marinate for 1 hour, or overnight in the fridge. Pull the pak choi leaves apart and put into a bowl. Slice the carrots into thin strips and baby corn in half lengthways. Add to the

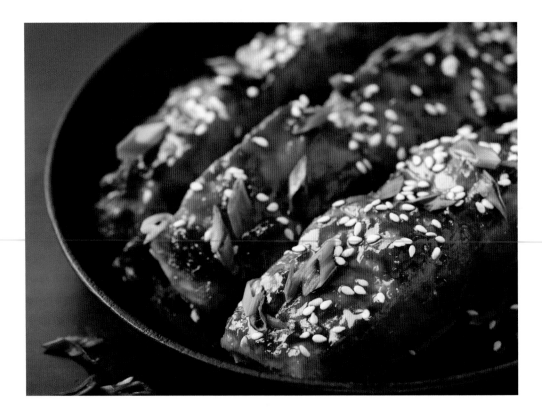

bowl. Using a potato peeler, shave the celery into strips and add to the bowl. Drizzle over the sesame oil and toss well. Heat a frying or griddle pan until hot. Remove salmon from marinade and then put skin-side down into the pan. Cook for 4 mins on each side, spooning over any extra marinade. Place the salmon fillets on a bed of the sesame oil veggies and serve with a wedge of lemon.

Per serving: cals 432 | fat 25 g | sat fat 4 g | protein 32 g

Turkey burgers with lemon and mint (serves 4)

• 450 g/ 1 lb minced turkey • ½ small onion, grated • Zest and juice of 1 lemon • 1 garlic clove, finely chopped • 3 tbsps mint, chopped • Pinch of dried chilli flakes • Beaten egg white

Method

In a bowl, combine all the above ingredients, mix and season. Shape into 8 burgers about 2 cm thick. Cover and leave in the fridge for at least an hour. Heat a griddle or frying pan and cook for 4–5 minutes each side. Serve with a mixed salad and low-fat mayonnaise.

Per serving: cals 182 | fat 3 g | sat fat 0.9 g | protein 28 g

Stir-fried chicken and red pepper (serves 2)

• 3 tbsps olive oil • 2 garlic cloves, sliced thinly • 1 small red pepper, deseeded and thinly sliced • 2 chicken breasts, cut into strips • 2 tbsps soy sauce • 100 g/3½ oz bag baby spinach leaves

Method

Heat a wok, add 2 tbsps of the olive oil and the garlic. Stir-fry until turning golden, then spoon onto kitchen paper to drain. Add the pepper and stir-fry for 1 min until slightly softened, then spoon out and set aside. Add the remaining tbsp of oil, add the chicken and stir-fry for another 5 minutes. Add the soy sauce and the spinach and stir-fry until it begins to wilt. Return the peppers and garlic to the wok and serve.

Per serving: cals 270 | fat 18 g | sat fat 3 g | protein 25 g

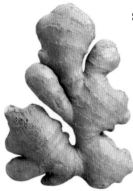

Salmon fillet and ginger (serves 2)

• 2 x 150 g/5¼ oz salmon steaks • 1cm piece root ginger, grated • 2 spring onions, finely sliced • Soy sauce, to season • Handful of coriander leaves • Basmati rice, steamed (not in calorie count)

Method

Heat the oven to 200°C/390°F/Gas Mark 6. Put each salmon steak in the middle of a piece of baking parchment or foil. Put some ginger and spring onion on top of each and then add a few drops of soy sauce. Fold the parchment into parcels around the fish, put on a baking sheet and cook in the oven for 10 mins. Open the parcels, sprinkle over some coriander and serve with basmati rice.

Per serving: cals 283 | fat 18.5 g | sat fat 3 g | protein 28 g

Potato tortilla with salmon, spring onion and mint (serves 2)

• 6 Jersey Royal potatoes • 150ml/¼ pint milk • 1 x 200 g/7 oz salmon fillet • 1 bay leaf • 1 tbsp olive oil • 2–3 spring onions, chopped • 1 tbsp freshly chopped chives • 2 eggs, preferably organic • 50 g/1¾ oz Parmesan cheese, grated • Fresh mint leaves, to serve

Method

Cook the potatoes in boiling water for 8–10 mins until cooked but still firm. Drain and leave to cool then cut into thin slices. Meanwhile, bring the milk to a gentle simmer. Add the salmon and bay leaf and poach for about 5–6 mins. Drain on kitchen paper. Reserve 2tbsps of the poaching liquid. Preheat the grill to high. Heat the oil in a non-stick frying pan and fry the potatoes over a medium heat until lightly browned. Flake the salmon over the potatoes and scatter over the spring onions. Toss gently. Whisk the poaching liquid into the eggs along with the chives; pour into the pan. Cook for 3–4 mins, pulling the egg to the centre, until almost set. Sprinkle over the Parmesan and grill for 1–2 mins until golden and bubbling. Serve in wedges, garnished with mint leaves.

Per serving: cals 188 | fat 18 g | sat fat 3 g | protein 49 g

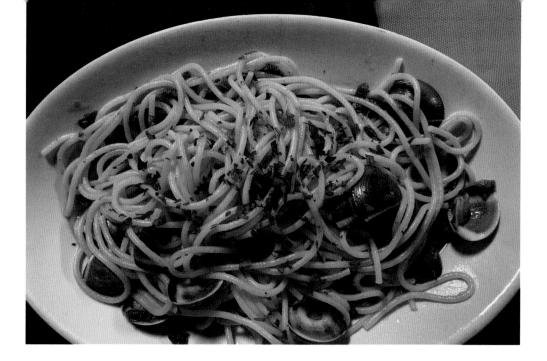

Spaghetti alle vongole (serves 4)

• 450 g/1 lb fresh clams in shells, washed • 2 garlic cloves, peeled and crushed • 1 small red chilli, deseeded and finely chopped • 400 g/14 oz tin of chopped tomatoes with herbs • 400 g/14 oz spaghetti • 2 tbsps olive oil • Freshly ground black pepper

Method

Discard any broken clams, and any that remain open when tapped. Put the rest into a large saucepan, cover and cook over a low heat for 3–4 mins, shaking the pan occasionally. Strain and reserve any juices. Discard any clams that remain closed and remove most of the meat from the shells, keeping a few intact for garnish. Heat 2 tbsps olive oil and fry the garlic and chilli for 1 min until soft. Add the tomatoes and 3 tbsps of the clam juice. Cook without a lid for 6–7 mins until thickened and dark red, stirring occasionally. Meanwhile, cook the spaghetti in boiling salted water for the time stated on the packet. Drain and add to the tomato sauce with the clam meat. Return to the heat for a few moments and then stir through. Season with black

Clams and chillies make for a luxurious accompaniment to spaghetti.

pepper and serve immediately, garnished with clam shells and a few fresh basil leaves.

Per serving: cals 255 | fat 7 g | sat fat 1 g | protein 19 g

Cod fillets with tomatoes and black olives (serves 4)
• 4 x 180 g/6½ oz boneless cod fillets • 175 g/6¼ oz black olives in olive oil, stones removed • 1 large onion, roughly chopped • 400 g/14 oz can chopped tomatoes • Salt and freshly ground black pepper • Handful of chopped parsley

Adding tomatoes and black olives makes a wonderfully tasty and nutritious way to serve cod.

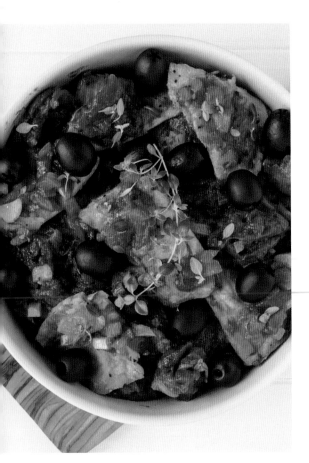

Method
Preheat the oven to 180°C/350°F/Gas Mark 4. Heat 1 tbsp of the oil from the olives in an ovenproof pan. Add the onion and stir well, leave to cook for a minute or 2, and then give it another good stir. Add the tomatoes and seasoning. Bring to the boil then add the olives. Put the fish, skin-side down, onto the sauce and drizzle over a splash more oil from the olive jar. Bake in the oven, uncovered, for 15 mins. Finish by sprinkling with chopped parsley and serve straight from the pan.

Per serving: cals 223 | fat 6 g | sat fat 1 g | protein 34 g

Stuffed peppers (serves 4)
• 4 red peppers, halved and seeded (leaves talks intact) • 225 g/8 oz cooked basmati rice • 1 small onion, chopped• 400 g/14 oz cherry tomatoes • 1 tbsp olive oil • 3 tbsps coriander, freshly chopped • 150 ml/¼ pint hot vegetable stock

Method
Heat the oil in a pan and gently fry the onion

for around 15 minutes. Add the
tomatoes and leave to simmer for
around 10 minutes. Stir in the cooked
rice and coriander, and then spoon the
mixture into the halved peppers. Place
the peppers in a roasting tin and pour
the stock around them. Bake for 30
mins (in preheated oven, 180°C/350°F/
Gas Mark 4) till tender.

Per serving: cals 208 | fat 5.2 g | sat
fat 1 g | protein 15 g

Mushroom frittata (serves 4)

• 300 g/10½ oz mixed mushrooms,
sliced (e.g. button, shiitake, chestnut)
• 6 medium eggs, beaten • 50 g/2 oz
watercress, chopped • 1 tbsp olive oil •
2tbsps thyme, freshly chopped • Zest
and juice of ½ lemon • Salt and freshly
ground black pepper

Method

Heat the olive oil in a large, deep
frying pan over a medium heat. Add
the mushrooms and thyme and stir-
fry for 5–6 minutes until starting
to soften and brown slightly. Stir in
the lemon zest and juice, leaving to bubble for around 1 minute. Now
lower the heat and preheat the grill. Add the watercress to the beaten
eggs, season to taste with the salt and pepper, and pour into the pan.
Cook for around 7–8 minutes until the sides and base are firm but the
centre is still soft. Then transfer the pan to the grill, cooking for 4–5
minutes until just set. Cut into wedges and serve with a green salad.

Per serving: cals 148 | fat 12 g | sat fat 3 g | protein 19 g

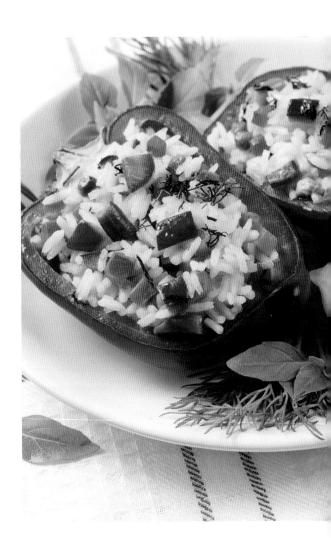

*Stuffed peppers
make a satisfying
meal and you can
vary the fillings
depending on what
you have available.*

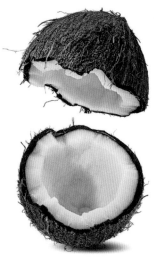

Coconut and ginger curried mussels (serves 4)

• 1.5 kg/ 3 lb 4 oz mussels • 2 tbsps olive oil • 3 shallots, chopped • 2 green chillies, deseeded and chopped • 4 cm/1½ in piece of root ginger, peeled and finely chopped • 1 tbsp mild curry paste • 1 x 400 ml/14 oz can coconut milk • Bunch of fresh coriander, chopped

Method

Scrub and de-beard the mussels, discarding any that remain open when given a sharp tap. Heat the olive oil in a very large saucepan and add the shallots, cooking for around 2–3 minutes until soft. Add the chillies and ginger and cook for a further minute. Add the mussels, cover, and cook for 3–4 minutes, shaking the pan occasionally, until the shells open. Stir the curry paste into the coconut milk and pour the mixture over the mussels. Cook for a further 3–4 minutes, then remove from the pan and discard any mussels with closed shells. Sprinkle over the chopped coriander and serve straight away.

Per serving: cals 361 | fat 13 g | sat fat 2 g | protein 19 g

Tasty chicken burgers (serves 4)

• 450 g minced chicken/1 lb • 1 small onion, finely chopped • 2 tsps tarragon, freshly chopped • 50 g/2 oz breadcrumbs • 2 large egg yolks

Method

Put the chicken into a bowl with the onion, tarragon, breadcrumbs and egg yolk. Mix well, then stir in 75 ml cold water and season. Divide into four portions and, using the back of a wet spoon, flatten each to a thickness of 2.5 cm. Cover and chill for 30 mins. Cook them under a hot grill or on a barbecue for about 6-7 mins, until cooked through.

Per serving: cals 105 |fat 2 g | sat fat 0.1 g | protein 19 g

Lemongrass beef and rice noodle salad (serves 4)

• 400 g/14 oz sirloin steak • 2 tbsps groundnut oil or vegetable oil • 1 small cucumber, peeled • 175 g/6¼ oz dried rice noodles• Drizzle of sesame oil • 1 small bunch coriander, stalks discarded and leaves left

whole • 2 spring onions, sliced • 250 g/9 oz pack cherry tomatoes,
cut in half

For the dressing • 1 red chilli, deseeded and finely chopped • 1 stalk
lemongrass, the bottom 7½ cm/3 in halved and very thinly sliced
• 1 tsp grated ginger • 1 small shallot, finely sliced • 2 tbsps
Thai fish sauce • 1 tbsp soft brown sugar • Juice of 1 lime

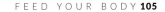

Method

Bring a large pan of water to the boil and season the steak.
Heat a griddle or frying pan with 2 tbsps groundnut or vegetable
oil until very hot. Cook the steak for 3–4 mins on either side until
seared on the outside and pink inside. Remove from the pan and leave
to rest for a few mins. Slice the steak thinly then transfer to a shallow
dish. Combine the dressing ingredients and stir until the sugar has
dissolved. Now spoon half the dressing over the still warm beef. Cut
the cucumber in half and run a vegetable peeler down the side so you
end up with thin ribbons. Discard the seedy core and set the ribbons
aside. Cook the noodles in the boiling water according to packet
instructions, then drain and rinse with cold water. Place the noodles
in a large bowl, drizzle a little sesame oil over the top and toss. Add
the beef and dressing and stir. Throw in the coriander, spring onions,
cucumber and tomatoes with the remaining dressing and toss again.
Per serving: cals 422 | fat 14 g | sat fat 4 g | protein 35 g

Thai chicken broth (serves 4)

• 200 g/7oz cooked chicken • 1–2 tbsps medium curry paste • 200ml
reduced-fat coconut milk • 600ml/1 pint vegetable stock • 2 pak choi,
chopped • Handful of sugar snap peas • 4 spring onions, chopped

Method

Heat the curry paste in a pan, then add the coconut milk and stock.
Bring to the boil. Then add the chicken, pak choi, sugar snap peas and
spring onion. Simmer for 2–3 mins. Serve in warmed bowls.
Per serving: cals 110 | fat 4 g | sat fat 0.1 g | protein 17 g

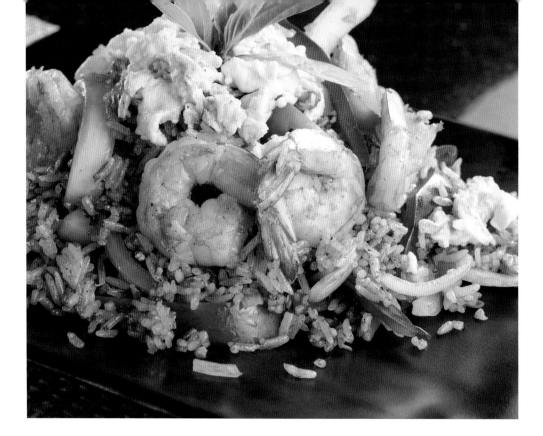

Juicy prawns add protein to tasty fried rice.

Fried rice with prawns (serves 4)

• 150 g/7 oz cooked basmati rice • 2 tbsps sesame oil • 3 eggs, lightly beaten • 250 g/5¼ oz cooked peas • 250 g/9 oz cooked, peeled prawns

Method

Heat 1 tsp of oil in an omelette pan, pour in half the beaten egg, tilting the pan for about 1 min until egg is set. Put omelette onto a warm plate. Repeat with the remaining egg to make another omelette. Again keep warm. Add the remaining oil to the pan and stir in the rice and peas until warmed through. Then stir in the prawns. Roll up the omelettes and chop into three. Add the chopped omelette to the rice and peas and cook for 1–2 mins until heated through. Divide the rice among four warmed bowls and top with the omelette.

Per serving: cals 328 | fat 11 g |s at fat 2 g | protein 21 g

Tuna Niçoise (serves 4)

• 400 g/14 oz tuna steaks • 200 g/7 oz green beans • 4 free-range eggs, preferably organic • 100 g/3½ oz black olives, stoned • 200 g/7 oz cherry tomatoes, halved • 8 anchovy fillets, chopped (optional) • Small bunch parsley, chopped to garnish

Method

Season the tuna with salt and pepper, heat a griddle pan and cook it over a high heat for 2 minutes on each side, so it remains rare on the inside. (Cook for longer if you prefer.) Meanwhile cook the green beans in boiling water for 2 minutes then drain under cold water. Put the eggs into gently boiling water and cook for 3 minutes, drain and place under cold running water to cool down quickly. Arrange the beans, olives and tomatoes on 4 plates. Break the tuna into pieces and toss over. Peel the eggs (they should still be soft in the middle) and add to the salad. Sprinkle over the anchovies, if using. Garnish with parsley and a lemon quarter and drizzle with olive oil.

Per serving: cals 266 | fat 13 g | sat fat 4 g | protein 25 g

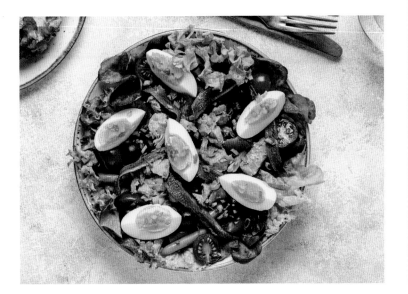

A super-healthy version of a favourite Niçoise salad.

HORMONAL HELP

Harmonise your hormones with these potent balancing foods

Of all the changes your body undergoes during midlife, the decline in oestrogen is perhaps the most profound. This can begin as soon as our late thirties. It affects not only body fat distribution — it tends to accumulate around the middle — but can also lead to poor sleep, lower energy, mood swings and hot flushes. Our hormonal, or endocrine, system is highly complex and there is no one food or supplement that can directly affect it, so it's best to eat a varied diet. However, there are certain foods that support hormone production and function.

PHYTOESTROGENS

These are plant chemicals that act like oestrogen in your body and are thought to lower rates of certain cancers, cardiovascular problems, and menopausal symptoms. Soya beans are the richest food source of phytoestrogens (buy organic, non-GMO soy), but they are also found in flaxseeds, dried fruit, sesame seeds, garlic, and bean sprouts.

LEAN PROTEIN

Amino acids found in lean protein are the building blocks of hormones, so it is important to eat plenty of good-quality protein. Eggs, fish, and lean meats are all excellent sources, while plant-based sources include quinoa, oats, beans, lentils and nuts. Tryptophan is an amino acid used in the production of serotonin, the 'feel-good' hormone. It plays a key role in regulating mood, sleep and appetite. You can find it in eggs, turkey, cottage cheese, seeds and nuts.

HEALTHY FATS

Generally found in veg, nuts, seeds and fish, healthy fats are crucial for hormone production. When cooking, stick to oils high in monounsaturates such as olive or organic rapeseed. Omega-3 supports oestrogen production so eat lots of oily fish.

TOP THREE HORMONE HELPERS

BROCCOLI contains the phytochemical Indole-3-Carbinol (I3C), which increases oestrogen metabolism. Try roasting it in the oven with garlic, olive oil and lemon juice – the garlic is high in phytoestrogens too.

SOY, including miso (below), edamame, tempeh and fermented tofu, are rich in isoflavones, a type of phytoestrogen, and are thought to be one of the reasons for a low incidence of menopausal symptoms among Japanese women. You can buy frozen edamame beans in most supermarkets, and they make a great change from frozen peas.

AVOCADOS are rich in healthy monounsaturated fats. As a change from avo toast, try making a beautifully creamy smoothie by blending avocado, banana, a little milk and a touch of cinnamon. Delicious.

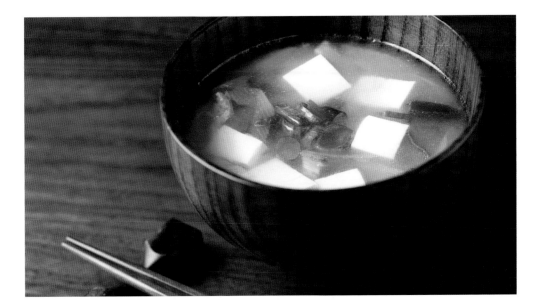

HEALTHY GUT

Treat your gut and your whole body will thank you for it

FEED YOUR GOOD BUGS WITH OATS
They tend to get less attention, but prebiotics are just as important as probiotics, as they feed the friendly flora in your large intestine. Oats are a great source of prebiotic fibre – go for the least refined possible, so organic steel-cut rather than microwave sachets.

MAKE A BEELINE FOR BANANAS
Though high in fruit sugar, bananas also contain prebiotic fibres to nourish the 'good' bacteria. What's more, if you eat over-ripe bananas, you're benefiting from a substance called Tumor Necrosis Factor (TNF), which has been found to destroy cancerous tumours.

BOLSTER WITH BONE BROTH
Made using animal bones – usually from cows, chickens or fish – this wholesome, warming elixir has been championed for its healing powers. Bone broth contains collagen and amino acids proline and glycine, which can help to heal and repair a damaged gut lining – often thought to be the cause behind autoimmune conditions. Broth is also super-easy to digest.

HEAL WITH COCONUT
Healthy fats in moderation are easy on your gut and promote healing. The medium-chain fatty acids in coconuts are easier to digest than other fats so work wonders if your gut is a little out of sync. They also have antifungal properties, to help reduce bad bacteria in your system.

GET A BOOST FROM BROCCOLI
Cruciferous vegetables, such as broccoli, cabbage and Brussels sprouts,

contain compounds called indole glucosinolates. When broken down in your stomach, they help strengthen your immune system and balance your gut flora (the live bacteria). Broccoli's sulphur-containing compounds also help detoxify and fight inflammation.

GO CRAZY FOR KEFIR

Kefir is a cultured, fermented milk drink with a tart, sour taste and it's a fantastic source of probiotics. Kefir contains numerous types of lactic acid bacteria, which help to stop harmful bacteria setting up camp in your gut.

TRY TRADITIONAL KIMCHI

This Korean fermented cabbage not only helps improve your gut's natural pH level by making it more acidic – a good thing! – but also boosts the number of healthy bacteria that aid digestion. We believe regular consumption of kimchi may also prevent the growth of H.pylori, a type of bacteria that can lead to stomach problems, including ulcers.

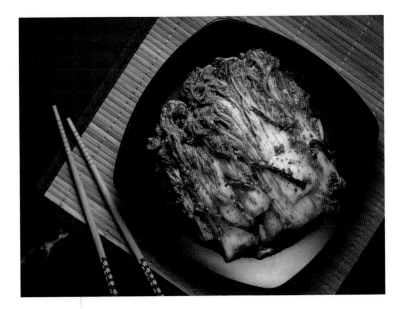

Try delicious kimchi to aid digestion.

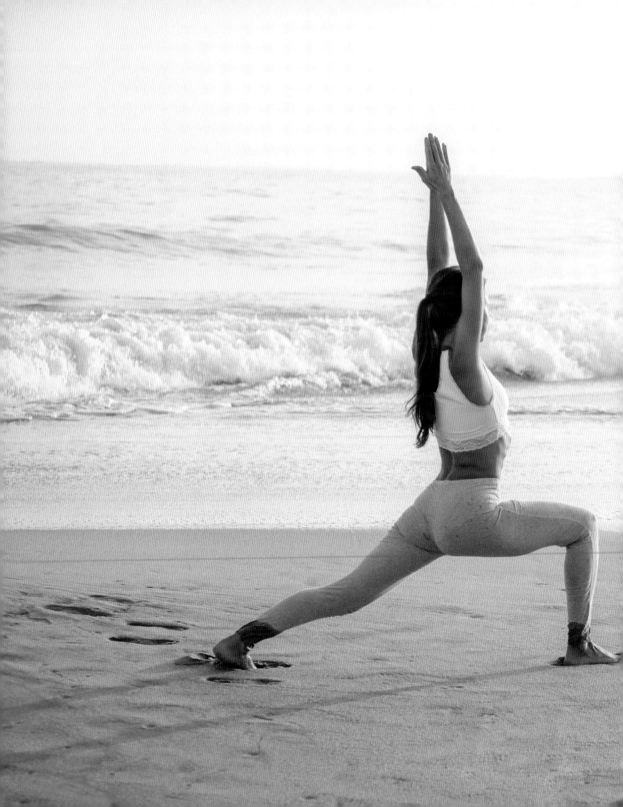

HOW TO RELAX WITH YOGA

Yoga is a fantastic way to relax and stretch out muscles that may have been tightened by other exercise. Its meditative properties are great for concentration and relieving stress.

YOGA FOR LIFE

Stay fit and healthy with yoga

Yoga really is a great all-rounder when it comes to staying fit for life. Research has shown that people who practise yoga regularly are thinner than their non-practising counterparts, have better appetite control and fewer cravings as well as better postural stability. Studies show that regular yoga over time leads to a lower body mass index (BMI), a lowered waist-to-hip ratio and lower body fat levels. Perhaps best of all, yoga has been shown to not only make our bodies look better, with longer, leaner muscles, but also to change the way we feel towards our bodies. Let's

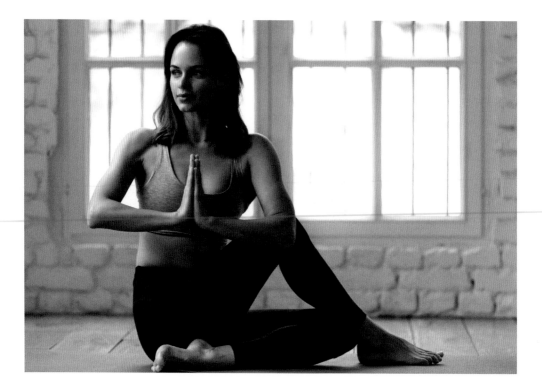

take a look at the ways yoga practice helps us achieve body transformation in more detail.

MORE MINDFUL EATING

Literally translated, yoga means 'union' of the mind and body. So many of our food and overeating issues today have come from being out of touch with what our bodies really need and what we're really feeling, so we use food as a crutch and comfort or an escape from difficult emotions. In fact, a study by A.R. Kristal at the Fred Hutchinson Cancer Research Center in Seattle, USA, used a mindful eating scale and found that people who practise yoga were more likely to eat mindfully – they ate when they were hungry and not because they were bored. By putting us back in touch with the needs of our minds and bodies, making us more mindful of our emotions, we're happier to 'just sit' with those more painful feelings, knowing they will pass. In this way, weight loss becomes a by-product of yoga's ability to make us healthier and more whole in both body and mind.

LESS STRESS-RELATED FAT

When it comes to weight, authorities are fond of telling us it's all about burning off more than we consume. But research is suggesting that hormonal imbalances play a key part in weight – especially that stubborn spare tyre around the middle – in particular elevated levels of the hormone cortisol, which is secreted by the adrenal glands in response to stress (two tiny glands that sit above your kidneys). Cortisol is the hormone that wakes us up and gets us motivated in the mornings. But when we have too much from constantly being under stress, it can cause an increase in appetite and constant cravings, a loss of muscle mass, decreased libido and an accumulation of fat around the middle. A study

CHECK LIST

WHAT YOGA can do for your body
- Lowers stress hormones which helps to shift your belly fat
- Balances your appetite
- Reduces emotional eating
- Helps stop sweet cravings
- Helps you sleep, which can balance appetite-regulating hormones
- Builds your muscles, which increases metabolism
- May shift cellulite by helping to clear toxins
- Lengthens your muscles

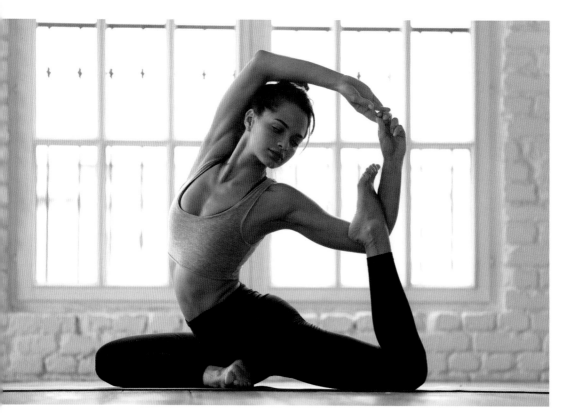

by Yale University in the US found that even slim women were more likely to have excess abdominal fat if they felt stressed regularly. That's because abdominal fat has more cortisol receptors than fat elsewhere in the body. Other tell-tale signs of high cortisol include waking in the small hours as your body prepares to fight a perceived threat. Interestingly, while cardiovascular exercise is important for weight control, going too hard and for too long can increase production of stress hormones and lead to an inability to lose weight. Regular yoga practice reduces stress hormones in the body and primes your organs' repair systems so your entire endocrine system is more balanced. This includes thyroid and sex hormones as well as insulin, imbalances of which can also affect weight.

DE-STRESSSING AND SLIMMING

Yoga is a great de-stressing practice to do at least once or twice a week (or more often– it's great in the evenings before bed). This is because although most people think only fast, flowing yoga is good for weight loss, new research shows otherwise. Researchers divided overweight women into two groups. One group took regular restorative yoga sessions and the other did stretching sessions. Both groups did this twice a week for 12 weeks, then twice a month for six months and finally once a month for three months. According to the results of the study, published in the *American Journal of Managed Care*, the restorative yoga group lost significantly more subcutaneous fat – that's the kind of fat directly under your skin – and kept it off for longer than the stretching group.

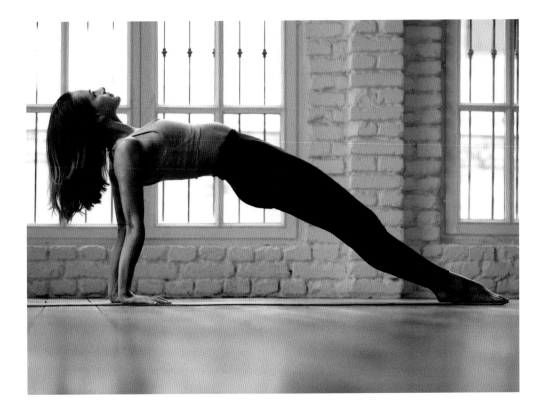

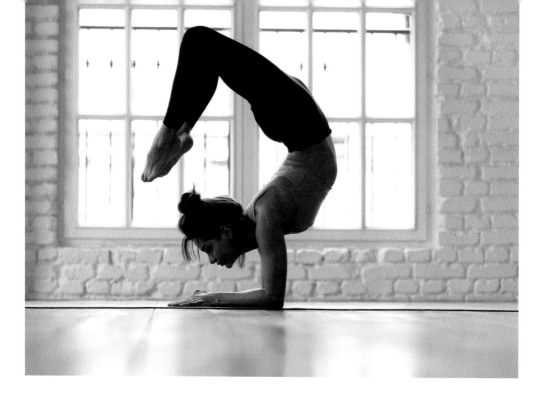

FASTER METABOLISM

From around the age of 30, your metabolic rate decreases by about five per cent per decade. But by increasing strength in your body, you can combat this process and help increase your natural metabolic speed. Here's how: at rest, your body uses around 35 calories to maintain a pound of muscle each day and only two calories to sustain a pound of fat. By simply adding 2–4 lb (1–2 kg) of muscle to your body, you could burn 100 extra calories a day, even when you are doing nothing. This is because muscle has a much higher metabolic rate than fat, so with more muscle you'll burn more calories, even when you're not exercising. So you can maintain a good metabolism as you get older. Yoga contributes to this equation because it uses your own bodyweight to build strength. For example, when you hold a pose, such as warrior or plank, you're working anaerobically (without oxygen) and, as a result, building your body's strength through the resistance created between your body and the movement.

BRANCHES OF YOGA

AS YOGA GREW and spread through India, different branches developed relating to different forms of practice and appealing to different people. Hatha yoga, the kind we're focused on in the West, is just one.

HATHA YOGA

This is the physical form of yoga which has grown fastest in the West. Its purpose is to develop a strong, healthy body.

BHAKTI YOGA

It uses devotional practices that involve chanting, singing and dancing. Its mission is to worship the divine.

JNANA YOGA

The most intellectual of the yoga types, it focuses on studying yoga and controlling the mind towards self-awareness.

KARMA YOGA

This involves selfless work or service for others as a path to the divine.

MANTRA YOGA

Uses the hearing sense to focus the mind in the form of mantras, sounds or music.

RAJA YOGA

It uses meditation to cultivate mind control.

TANTRA YOGA

It emphasises pleasure and ecstasy in all of life's experiences – both good and those we might consider bad or challenging – to release the body's energy and power.

LONGER, LEANER MUSCLES: CELLULITE FIX

It's not yet proven, but if you've ever wondered how yoga instructors' bodies look so smooth and cellulite-free, it could be down to their practice. The intense stretching aspect of yoga not only creates longer, leaner and more defined muscles, it also promotes circulation, which some believe might help flush out the areas in the bottom and thighs where toxins and cellulite reside. Each of our circuits is specifically designed to combine strengthening and stretching of your muscles so the end result is a stronger, leaner and longer look.

AND RELAX ...

Stretching, relaxation and recovery play an important role in staying in tip top form, which is where yoga really comes into its own ...

When we're overtired or stressed we can be too wired to get to sleep, which is the thing we need most! In yoga, we're encouraged to honour our body's fatigue through postures that work the circulatory, endocrine and nervous systems in a way that encourages and gently coaxes the mind and limbs into deep relaxation. That rejuvenating and rebuilding effect sweeps up the damage caused by stress, so we encourage you to do this circuit at least once a week. It's also the perfect antidote to a busy day, to help encourage a deep and restful sleep.

CHILD'S POSE – BALASANA

BENEFITS: Great for relieving bloating or gas. Stretches and soothes the lower back and upper body, opens the hips. Lowers heart rate and is deeply soothing. Great if you're feeling panicky.

Kneel with legs tucked under, knees apart, pelvis resting on your shins and tops of the feet on the floor. Inhale. Place a bolster or two thick pillows lengthways between your knees. Exhale and move your torso forward so it drapes onto the bolster and your head turns to one side to rest. Relax your arms by the sides of the bolster, or make a pillow for your head by placing one flat palm on top of the other on the bolster and resting your forehead on your hands. Relax your head and neck and feel your torso sink down into the bolster. Breathe slowly and deeply for one to five minutes, directing your breath into the back ribs. Relax the entire torso on each exhalation.

VARIATION: Try removing the bolster and doing the pose with your head resting on a block or book about five centimetres high. Rest your

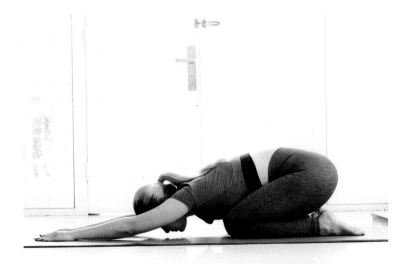

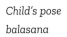

Child's pose
balasana

head on it at the point of your third eye. Relax into the posture for 20–24 breaths for a deeply relaxing experience.

EXTENDED MOUNTAIN POSE, STRETCHING TO SIDE – URDHVA HASTASANA

BENEFITS: Encourages deeper breathing. Deeply stretches the arms and oblique muscles.

Begin in mountain pose, centring your weight on all four corners of your feet, focusing on your breath. Turn palms outward, inhale and lift your arms out to your sides and up towards the ceiling, stopping when they're parallel. Reach up through your hands without compressing your neck and keeping your shoulders down. Take five breaths. On an exhalation, reach both arms over to the left, feeling a stretch in the right side of your body; don't let your torso come forward. This is a side stretch so it's better to move a little to the side than a lot. Take hold of your right wrist with the left hand. Take five breaths. Repeat on the other side. Do the pose twice on each side.

Extended mountain pose, stretching to side – Urdhva hastasana.

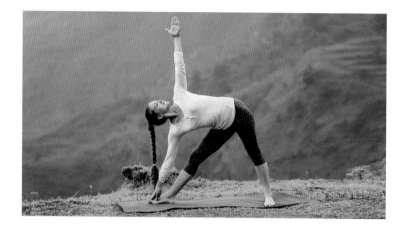

TIP: As you stretch to the right, press your left foot into the floor, and vice versa, for a deeper stretch. You can tug a little with the holding hand but make sure the body stays looking forward.

STANDING FORWARD BEND – UTTANASANA

BENEFITS: Deeply relaxing for the mind and relieves tiredness. Strengthens and stretches your hamstrings, tones your spine.

From mountain pose, inhale and lift your arms up over your head. Exhale, bend your knees slightly and fold forward from your hips (not your waist) and relax your upper body towards the floor. Fold your arms, holding each elbow with the opposite hand, and let your head hang loosely. Bend your knees a little deeper so your torso is resting on the tops of your thighs. Take 20 breaths. On an inhalation, slowly roll upwards, rounding the spine, imagining you're stacking one verterbra over the other until your spine is straight.

TIP: For a super-relaxing tension reliever, really let go of the whole upper body in this pose, bending your knees as deeply as you need to. It feels great to shake your head as if you're saying 'no' five times and then to nod it as though you're saying 'yes' another five times.

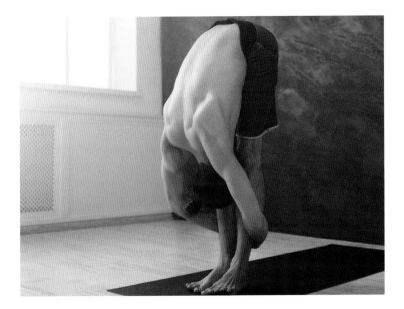

*Standing
forward bend —
uttanasana.*

RELAXING SQUAT – MALASANA

BENEFITS: Releases tension in the shoulders and hips (great after sitting all day).

Start in mountain pose, feet hip-distance apart and slightly turned out and parallel. Inhale and place hands in prayer position. Exhale and bend your knees as you come forward from your hips, as though trying to sit in a chair. Keeping your chest and shoulders open and knees apart, lower your hips down further until your torso is between your knees. Separate your feet as much as you need to in order to keep your heels on the floor (you may need to turn them out a little more) and sink your heels into the floor. Place your hands on the floor in front of you, letting your torso and head hang forward for 15–20 breaths. To come out, lower your body onto all fours.

VARIATION: If your heels are coming off the floor, place a block under each heel.

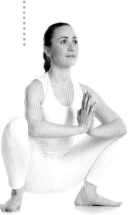

RECLINING HEAD-TO-TOE SEQUENCE – SUPTA PADANGUSTHASANA

BENEFITS: Deeply stretches the hamstrings, groin and inner thighs. Promotes deep relaxation and sleep.

Lie flat. Bend your left knee and hug it to your chest with your arms. Take five breaths here. Inhale and straighten your left leg, holding your big toe with your left fingers (if you can't reach, take your shin with both hands).

Keep your shoulders down and relaxed. Ensure your straight right leg remains engaged and rotating inwards, knee facing up, toes pointing up and heel flexing forward. Beginners: If this feels strained and causes the lower back to lift off the floor, bend your right knee and place your foot flat on the floor. Take five deep breaths. Now, externally rotate your left leg so your toes point out to the side. Slowly lower your leg to the left side as far as is comfortable without your right leg tipping over.

Relax your shoulders and neck and keep the lower leg engaged. Keep the right hip down (it will want to rise!). You can gently guide the hip down with the right hand. Take five breaths. Bring the left leg back to the centre and gently release. Repeat on the other side. Do the sequence again on each side.

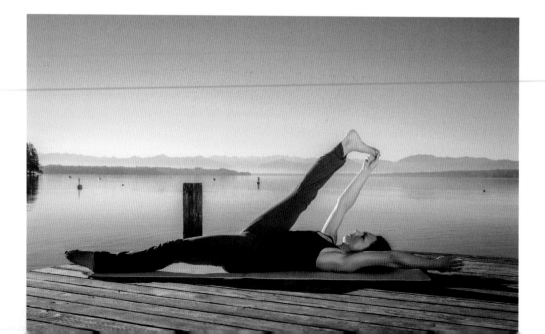

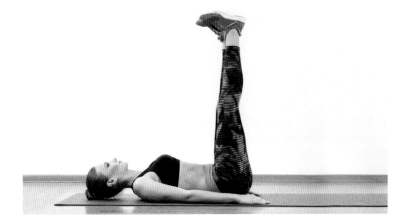

VARIATION: If it's straining you to hold your big toe in your fingers (you'll know this if your lower back is lifting off the floor more than a centimetre), take your shin instead, or use a strap or scarf wrapped around the ball of your foot.

TIP: Beginners can press the sole of the lying foot against a wall to help 'train' the leg to stay engaged.

SUPPORTED LEG LIFT

BENEFITS: Deeply relaxing for the entire body — the act of lifting your legs above your heart takes the pressure off your lower body resulting in a release of muscle tension.

Lie on your back. Bend your knees and gently lift your hips to place a brick flat under your lower back. Inhale and lift up your legs, keeping your knees bent gently towards your chest. Sway a little to massage the adrenal glands (located at the top of your kidneys). Really relax and take ten breaths. Now, on an inhalation, extend the legs up straight so your body is at a right angle. Take another ten breaths. To exit, bend and lower your legs so your feet touch the floor. Lift the hips and remove the block. Move straight into twisting adrenal massage (overleaf).

TWISTING ADRENAL MASSAGE

BENEFITS: Deeply relaxing and massaging for the adrenal glands. These two glands sit above each kidney and are responsible for the release of stress hormones.

Lie on your back. Bend your knees, inhale and lift up the legs, keeping your knees bent gently towards your chest. Keeping your knees and feet together, exhale and roll the lower body to the right, resting it a moment on the floor. Inhale and lift the lower body, exhaling as you ease it over to the left, resting a moment on the floor. Continue in this way for 10 breaths. Rest then repeat.

TIP: Taking the legs and feet from one side to the other should take one full breath, both inhalation and exhalation.

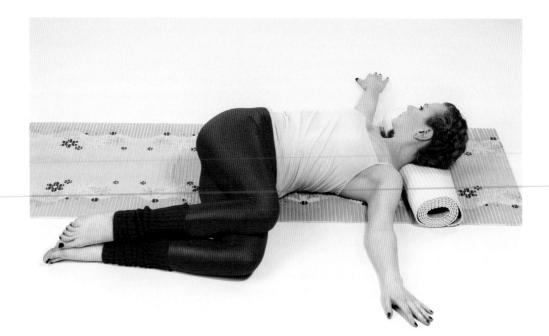

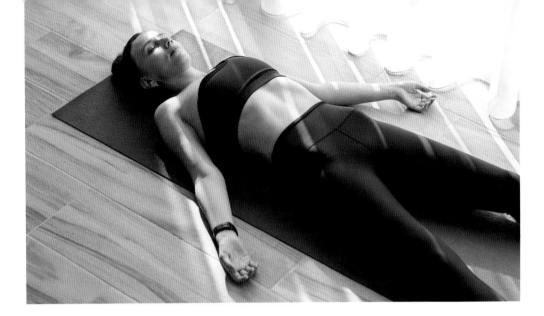

CORPSE – SAVASANA

BENEFITS: Stabilises your breathing, helps the muscles and mind relax and absorb the benefits of the practice.

Start seated on the floor. Bend your knees with feet hip-distance apart and hold the tops of your shins with your hands. Now lower your torso back by placing your forearms and palms onto the floor and leaning back on your elbows. Lower your torso to the floor one verterbra at a time until the back of your head rests on the floor. Turn your palms up to face the ceiling, arms about a foot away from your torso. Straighten your legs and let your feet relax out to the sides. Close your eyes, relax your whole body and focus on your breathing. Stay in this pose for up to five minutes.

VARIATIONS: If you have a tight lower back, place a bolster under your knees. If your neck is strained, place a block under the head. These modifications are extremely relaxing even if you don't have a sore back!

TIP: Your body temperature may drop in this pose so cover yourself with a blanket.